PRAISE FOR

On the Ledge

"This remarkable story of a woman's journey toward healing after a random, shocking accident takes us back in time into the home of an unusual family and the seminal event that shaped them all. In peeling back layers of trauma and revisiting key moments from her past, Turner comes to a new understanding of what it means to be a daughter, a mother, a woman, and a seeker of truth. This is a riveting story of courage and redemption. And dare I say that parts of it are very, very funny?"

—HOPE EDELMAN, #1 *New York Times* best-selling author of *Motherless Daughters* and *The AfterGrief*

"Her mother drank, her father went off his head in a way that made newspaper headlines, and four-year-old Amy Turner was left to pick up the pieces. Years later, after a devastating accident of her own, she begins to fit the shards of her upbringing together into an evocative portrait of a family whose secrets nearly buried them all. *On the Ledge* is sad, funny, wise, and lit with grace."

—TAD FRIEND, author of *In the Early Times*

"In her strong, gracious memoir, *On the Ledge,* Amy Turner deftly explores anxiety's pernicious cruelty. The flashes of insight into the toll that anxiety takes on the human spirit are never self-pitying, but constantly poignant and revealing."

—LOU ANN WALKER, author of *A Loss for Words: The Story of Deafness in a Family*

"In lyrical and vivid prose, Amy Turner reckons with her family secrets and how they dug their roots deep into her psyche. With trauma as the inciting force, Turner courageously comes to terms with her past and present, showing us how choosing to lean into the scars can reveal paths forward. *On the Ledge* is a compelling read, told with grace, vulnerability, and depth."

—RACHEL MICHELBERG, author of *Crash: How I Became a Reluctant Caregiver*

"Amy Turner artfully weaves the effects of her own near tragedy— she was run over by a truck, literally—into her lifelong search for the truth behind the very public rescue of her father from his precarious perch on the fifty-foot-high ledge of his hotel window. Through it all, her writing sparkles with insight, wit, self-deprecating humor, and subtle understatement. So skilled and honest is her prose that I felt myself no longer a mere reader, but a kindred soul in her struggles."

—TERRY MARSHALL, coauthor of *A Rendezvous to Remember*

"Absorbing, direct, humorous, horrific, *On the Ledge* explores the edge of madness as an artful memoir that also addresses two growing contemporary concerns: suicide and addiction. Timely, significant, well written, this is a courageous and engaging account, neither didactic nor sentimental, that belongs on school shelves as well as in the home."

—JOAN BAUM, host of NPR's *Baum on Books*

On

the

Ledge

_____

On the Ledge

A Memoir

Amy Turner

swp

SHE WRITES PRESS

Published 2022
Printed in the United States of America
Print ISBN: 978-1-64742-225-7
E-ISBN: 978-1-64742-226-4
Library of Congress Control Number: 2022904485

For information, address:
She Writes Press
1569 Solano Ave #546
Berkeley, CA 94707

She Writes Press is a division of SparkPoint Studio, LLC.

Book design by Stacey Aaronson

The author is grateful for permission to use excerpts from the following works:

From *Cheerful Money: Me, My Family, and the Last Days of Wasp Splendor* by Tad Friend, copyright © 2009. Reprinted by permission of Little, Brown, an imprint of Hachette Book Group, Inc.

"September 1, 1939," copyright ©1940 and renewed © 1968 by W. H. Auden; from SELECTED POEMS by W. H. Auden, edited by Edward Mendelson. Used by permission of Vintage Books, an imprint of Knopf Doubleday Publishing Group, a division of Penguin Random House LLC. All rights reserved.

"September 1, 1939," copyright © 1940 by W. H. Auden, renewed, reprinted by permission of Curtis Brown, Ltd. All rights reserved.

From "Little Gidding," from *Four Quartets* by T. S. Eliot, reprinted by permission of Faber and Faber Ltd., Publishers.

From "Little Gidding," from *Four Quartets* by T. S. Eliot, copyright © 1936 by Houghton Mifflin Harcourt Publishing Company, renewed 1964 by T. S. Eliot. Copyright © 1940, 1941, 1942 by T. S. Eliot, renewed 1968, 1969, 1970 by Esmé Valerie Eliot. Used by permission of HarperCollins Publishers.

"The Logical Song"
Words and music by Rick Davies and Roger Hodgson.
Copyright © 1979 by ALMO MUSIC CORP. and DELICATE MUSIC.
All rights controlled and administered by ALMO MUSIC CORP.
All rights reserved. Used by permission. Reprinted by permission of Hal Leonard LLC.

The author has made a good faith, diligent effort to identify and locate the copyright owners of the two photographs of her father standing on the ledge, but none could be found. The author wishes to thank photographer George Keeley, the *New Haven Register,* the Associated Press, and United Press International.

The author's family photo was taken by Robert Browning Baker.

Author's Note: The events and experiences described here are rendered as the author remembers them to the best of her ability. Names and identifying characteristics have been changed to protect the privacy of certain individuals.

For Ed,
Matthew, and Peter

We shall not cease from exploration
And the end of all our exploring
Will be to arrive where we started
And know the place for the first time.

—T. S. ELIOT, "Little Gidding"

TABLE OF CONTENTS

PROLOGUE

ON A COLD NOVEMBER MORNING IN 1957, AS
Yale students crossed the green to their first classes, hotel employees cleaned up breakfast dishes, and three priests went out for a walk, my father, pajama-clad and barefoot, climbed out on the ledge of his hotel window and threatened to jump. Some fifty feet below, the fire truck arrived. Three firemen cranked the extension ladder to the floor below him while others tried to gauge a jump's trajectory and positioned a circular net. Those in the growing crowd craned their necks to take in every moment of the unfolding drama. Soon, hundreds of people were staring up at him.

My mother, at home in Bronxville, New York, had awakened with an uneasy feeling—a low rumbling in her head, perhaps. She called my father's hotel room. When he didn't answer, she might have pictured him standing on the front porch of our house again, a fresh bloodstain on the front of his shirt. The injury had been superficial—from a penknife, it turned out—but having been self-inflicted, it was hard to forget. It's possible that she thought about pouring a scotch, but maybe the effect of last night's half bottle, or the memory of my father's confident smile as he boarded the train to New Haven that morning, reassured her.

Still getting no answer, my mother phoned my father's business colleague, who was staying in the room next to him, and asked that he check in on him. When he called back to say that her husband was standing on the hotel ledge, she called a close family friend, who drove her to New Haven.

Around the same time, the three priests out on their walk heard the commotion and hurried to the hotel. Father Keating and the prior dashed up to my father's room while Father Murphy remained on the sidewalk, ready to administer last rites, if necessary.

When my mother saw my father next, still in his pajamas and seated in a wheelchair at the hospital admissions desk, he just stared at her. She leaned forward and cupped her palms over his hands.

His knuckles, a range of bony peaks, did not soften.

She moved an inch closer. "Har . . . old?"

Still no response.

The doctor, glancing up from the counter where he was signing forms, answered for him, "Catatonic."

Later that afternoon, a New York City reporter conned his way into our house. Our maid, home alone and no doubt distracted by her four charges, didn't notice him pocketing a family photograph.

———

I was four and a half years old at the time, and all I knew for sure was what I could see—a father who sat behind a brown desk in my parents' bedroom, a mother who paused only to light a cigarette as she flashed by, a wrinkly-faced maid who yelled at us, a skinny black dog named Skeeter who ran away when I raised my arm, and an older sister who read me a book sometimes. I also had two younger brothers, but I hardly perceived them as separate from me. We were so close in age, we were like an amoeba whose edges could bulge out in three directions at once.

But it must have been soon after my father climbed onto the ledge when I began to sense something else coexisting in our house. If I'd known the word at four and a half, it might have been "trapdoor." I was certain that at any time and without warning, the floor could snap open, swallow one of us, and slam shut in a nanosecond. A trapdoor was invisible, of course, but I patrolled the house nonetheless, searching for warning signs—a retreat in my father's eyes, or a loosening in my mother's white-knuckled grip. In my family, loving or being loved was secondary. First, we had to avoid the trapdoors. And by the time I was sixteen and was finally told the truth about what had happened in 1957, I had been on high alert for a dozen years, the pattern so deeply ingrained that it would take another forty years to understand and undo it.

1

THE ACCIDENT

THE WEATHER'S INDECISION WAS CONTAGIOUS. AS SOON as my husband, Ed, and I rounded up some towels and chairs for the beach, it would rain, and then once we settled on an indoor chore, the sun would reappear.

The humidity—oppressive even by the standards of a July afternoon in East Hampton—was affecting us. By 2:30 p.m., the tension between us was as thick as the air.

It was my fault. I'd accepted a dinner invitation for us that evening knowing Ed wouldn't want to go. Annoyed about it this morning, he would've forgotten about it after a day at the beach. But with the event a few hours away and the beach out of the question, he had grown more irritated.

In 2010, after almost thirty years of marriage, I now knew better than to let our snits get out of hand. I also knew that pretending we were getting along at a dinner party with six couples would be far more unpleasant than apologizing again.

I took a deep breath, hoped my exhale wasn't audible, and tried to make my tone neutral. "Hey, what're you up to?"

Ed was carrying a bucket of water with a few rags—ripped, grayed undershirts—draped over its edges.

He cracked the front door and looked back over his shoulder at me, his face expressionless. Even at sixty (and despite some thinning hair and extra pounds), he still bore the good looks that had attracted me decades earlier.

"What does it look like? Going to wash my car."

"I'm sorry, Ed. I really am."

Ed put down the bucket. A few sudsy drops sloshed onto his flip-flopped foot. "I had a terrible week at work. I told you I have an important presentation on Monday. All I wanted to do was relax this weekend, and now I have to spend tonight with John and Alice, who you know drive me crazy. You should've asked me."

What he could've also pointed out, but generously didn't, was that I was on vacation from teaching seventh grade—that my summer, unlike his, was one long weekend.

"I know. I'm sorry . . . I wanted to see Sarah and Mark and didn't think you'd be so upset. Look, let me do you a favor. I'll get the dry cleaning." I glanced at my phone. "They close soon. I'm going to change my clothes and get going."

"Thanks, but don't bother. The traffic's going to be terrible. All the summer people will have left the beach and be driving around the village." The screen door clattered shut behind him.

Ed was hosing down his BMW, so he may not have heard me when I opened my car door ten minutes later. I should've said goodbye, but I was tallying our balance sheet of petty marital grievances.

I backed down the driveway—took care as I had a thousand times before (with more success at some times than others) to avoid the scraggly rhododendron that encroached at the narrowest point. We just needed space. We'd both be in better moods when I got back.

By the time I turned right onto Route 114, I needed the windshield wipers.

This wide, two-lane stretch of road, one of the few places in East Hampton where the speed limit exceeds forty miles per hour, is hardly bucolic. A couple of houses can be seen among the scrubby trees, but most are tucked away on intersecting dead-end streets, all but a few paved by now. But at the intersection with Stephen Hand's Path, a busy road itself, whose name recalls its origin in the 1660s as a twelve-foot-wide thoroughfare for "carts and oxen in yoake, [but] not . . . cattle . . . out of yoake," the view changes. The road slightly dips at the traffic light, and as it rises on the other side, I always feel a moment of lightness as I look out over the expanse of farm fields and sky, which on that day offered a palette of striated grays and blues.

I picked up Ed's shirts and suits from the dry cleaners, and as I left the store it looked like the clouds had disappeared for good. Hugging a thick pile of plastic-covered clothes to my chest with both arms, I stepped into the pedestrian crosswalk: no people, no cars. Then I noticed a dark blue pickup truck pulling out of the dead-end street almost directly across from me.

It wasn't one of those petite pickups that weekenders drive to try to pass themselves off as locals. This truck was large and sitting up high like it had important business to take care of.

Surely the driver had seen me standing in a marked crosswalk, its sign clearly visible atop a pedestal that said, "Stop for Pedestrians." I took another step.

By now the truck was turning into my lane. If the windshield weren't shaded, I could have seen the driver's face. I was surprised but not scared. He *had* to be seeing me. I was six feet in front of him, in broad daylight.

He can't possibly mow me down . . . What? He's accelerating. I can almost touch the windshield. Oh God. It can't be. He's going to hit me. I'm going to die. I squeezed the dry cleaning.

I froze in a combination of terror and resignation, yet—and I would be ashamed to admit this later—in that moment I also felt a fleeting sense of relief, even freedom. I could finally let go, release the fear I had spent a lifetime trying to contain.

The hood plowed into me at shoulder level with a thud so heavy and determined it seemed propelled like the earth itself. I felt rather than heard the sound: a deep rumbling like some tectonic plate had shifted below. I could feel the pounding on the left side of my chest and shoulder, but before the pain registered, I was thrown back and my head crashed onto the pavement. It bounced, but without the give of a ball, and when it hit the street again, it was with the hardness of a boulder dropping onto concrete.

Some part of me knew this impact should hurt like hell and that my brain might have been splattered on the street, but I felt fiery pain for only a split second.

I heard a whooshing sound and had the sensation of moving in an arc. I either lost consciousness or just couldn't think.

All motion stopped. I was alone in a dark silence, perfectly quiet except for the strangely comforting sound of the engine blowing hot air on me. My first thought was utter surprise—as though the screen had suddenly gone dark in the middle of a movie and the audience had been asked to go home.

This can't possibly be it. No warning, not even a hint. No chance to say goodbye?

I scanned the black screen.

Ed will be okay, I thought. *He knows I love him, and by now we've said it all. But the boys? Matthew and Peter.* A sob began to form, but it froze at the bottom of my throat.

I couldn't believe I wouldn't see my sons again, say goodbye, hug them . . .

Others might see their pasts flash by in similar situations, but I flipped forward—through future family photographs and events that had yet to pass: graduations, weddings, wives, grandchildren. But it was too hard to keep making it up, and when the pictures faded, I felt the urge to scream. I would scream myself back into this life. Scream so Matt and Peter could hear me. Scream that I loved them, that I'd made so many mistakes, that I was so, so sorry, that I wished I'd been a better mother.

But I couldn't scream; I couldn't even breathe. The plastic-covered clothes I'd been carrying were covering my face. For a second, I noted the irony. I'd just been hit by a truck, but I was going to die suffocating on my dry cleaning.

My brain begged my arms to remove the plastic, but they just lay there, unresponsive. My legs wouldn't move either. Paralyzed. I gasped reflexively. Stupid idea. It only sucked the plastic deeper into my throat. *Stop panicking,* I yelled at myself, *you'll choke even more—think of something!* I tried to force the plastic out with a cough, but it was too far down. The pressure in my head was getting unbearable. I was going to drown.

Suddenly, fingers were rubbing the roof of my mouth, and in a second I could breathe. With the air came sounds and sight and, within me, a flood of love and gratitude.

A car door slammed. "Oh God, I'm so sorry . . ."

I looked up. Through a foggy haze, I saw a tall, slim young man with blond hair. Was it Matt?

"Don't worry, I'm alive—I'm alive—I'll be okay," I told him.

I wanted to hug him and let him know that I forgave him for this accident, forgave him for everything. That all that matters in this world is how we love, and I loved him no matter what. I could move my arm now, but a hug meant getting up. So instead I reached for whatever I could touch—the outside of his calf, it turned out—and patted it.

As I looked up at him, the picture cleared a little. I was forgiving a stranger.

A cop appeared next to him. "We're going to get the truck off you. Don't move, because your foot is touching the tire."

I couldn't move, so I was sure this wouldn't be a problem, but the thought scared me even more than I already was. Desperate to find a joke that might distract me, I said, "Okay, as long as you don't let the driver do it."

The ignition started, and then the heat was off my face. First, the trees came into view—slim, impossibly tall, as though they were growing under my gaze. And then came the promises: *I'm never going to obsess about my weight again. I'm never going to pressure my children. I'll never say I feel like I got hit by a truck when all I mean is that I'm tired. I'll live one day at a time. I won't carry a grudge. I'll just love.*

God, how liberating.

Awash in those feelings of gratitude and acceptance, I wasn't prepared for fear to come roaring in: *What if I can't walk? What if I'm paralyzed? What if I'm brain-damaged?* To stop this stream of questions, I started a monologue of sorts. "I'm a mom," I said out loud, managing just a few words at a time. "I have . . . two sons, a husband . . . teach at Springs, co-president of the union. I . . . can't lie here . . . We have a . . . contract to negotiate . . ."

I knew what I was saying was absurd, but I was determined

to convince the paramedics that I was ready to return to life as usual. If I could recite my to-do list, maybe they would let me do it. They needed to identify me, but I couldn't think of my name. Rather than acknowledge this potential evidence of brain damage, I directed them to what I could remember. "Tell the dry cleaners . . . they know me . . . I'm the one with the squirrel . . ."

For me, the best defense is always humor. I tried to speak loud enough to block out the worried conversation of the people crouched around me and tell the story of the time I unwittingly dropped off a squirrel along with my clothes to be drycleaned. It seemed impossible to me that a squirrel would have made my sweater its temporary home and then have had the survival instinct to make it all the way to the dry cleaners and wait to hop out until what it perceived to be the opportune time.

It was just as well that a man with a deep, booming voice shut me up. "We know who you are. We remember the story." I learned later that it was George, the owner of the dry cleaners and, lucky for me, the best EMT on the East End. God knows he was probably sick of the story.

They tried to move me, but I didn't want to know what had happened to the back of my head—to hear that I had a gaping wound, or that my brains had spilled onto the sidewalk. Each time they tried, I yelled that I was going to throw up or that my head was going to burst. Men hunched by my head on my left side. I knew they were men because of their low voices.

"Where does your head hurt?" one of them asked.

Stupid fucking question. It just bounced on concrete. An image of a melon smashed on pavement came to mind.

Stupid question, but I couldn't remember the words "left" or "right." I could only picture the truck.

"Driver's side, back seat."

I hadn't meant to be funny, but they laughed.

"You mean, left side of your head toward the back?" one asked, translating.

"Yeah." I could feel a burning back there and a buzzing throughout my body, as if the impact had tripped an electrical switch. The sensations didn't seem to have a physical origin; rather, they seemed to be springing from my thoughts, from my imagining what it must feel like to be hit by a truck.

"Okay, but we really have to lift your head. We've got to see what's going on back there."

I squeezed my eyes shut. I was not going to do it. I did not want to know.

And then from my right side, away from the men, came a woman's voice—a soothing Irish lilt—saying, "Please, dear, we really must bandage you."

I didn't want to say no to someone whose voice was so gentle, loving, and concerned. I searched my brain for a thought, an image, a something that might give me the courage to lift my head, and found myself picturing the posters in my seventh-grade social studies classroom. I closed my eyes and said, or probably mumbled, with as much determination as I could muster, "Okay, I'll do it—I'm at Valley Forge. George Washington needs me; I can handle it."

A few moments later, with white gauze around my forehead, I probably looked like the fife player in that iconic trio of bedraggled patriots marching off to war.

They managed to get me into a neck and body brace and

lift me into the ambulance. Then it dawned on me that Ed hadn't arrived yet. "Where's my husband?"

"We called him. He'll meet you at the airport. You're a head trauma. You have to go to Stony Brook."

The Irish angel began to say goodbye, and I practically commanded her to come with me. "I need your voice—I'm too scared, please, you're the only one who makes me feel better."

Even at the time, my unequivocal admission of neediness surprised me. I would later learn that she was just someone who had been passing by. God knows what else she had on her plate for that day; it certainly wasn't to minister to a voluble crash victim. I begged her, though, and she came with me to the airport.

I don't remember anything of the ten-minute ride, not even the sound of the siren. Perhaps comforted by the Irish woman at my side and the thought of seeing Ed soon, I was relaxed enough to slip into semiconsciousness.

———

At the airport, the ambulance doors opened, and a face appeared about six inches from mine. It was huge, and then it shrunk to the size of a little boy's, and finally Ed came into focus.

Relief yielded to fear. I'm known to be absentminded, and I'd caused him enough grief in our marriage. Now he had to spend the weekend in the hospital with me. "It wasn't my fault. I swear. He just hit me. I'm so sorry."

I could tell from Ed's expression that it hadn't occurred to him to hold me responsible. But he didn't have to. Ever since childhood I'd been holding myself responsible for events outside my control. My father's mental state. The possibility that my mother would drink again. My children's tears. And now an oncoming truck.

In my mental fog, I'd forgotten about the Irish angel sitting next to me. Later, Ed told me he'd assumed she was an EMT. When he subsequently overheard her asking for a ride into town, he realized his mistake and wondered who she was.

Ed's face kept going in and out of focus, as though I were adjusting a lens. I heard someone telling him what had happened and what was wrong with me. Ed, of course, was desperate to hear the information; I was desperate not to. I started making buzzing sounds as loud as I could to drown out their conversation. Ed begged me to stop, but in a minute I didn't need to buzz because something else was doing a much better job at it—the waiting helicopter.

Now that Ed was there, I felt safe for the first time since the truck hit me. When they told me he couldn't come with me on the flight, I couldn't find the words. How was it possible to be so afraid and hurt and yet not be allowed to be with the one person you needed?

As they pulled me out of the ambulance, the heavens opened and the rain came down in sheets. They shielded my face with a blanket. It was so heavy that it blocked out the light and pressed down into my mouth. I felt like I was once again under the truck with the plastic dry-cleaning bag on top of me. I couldn't breathe. In a state of anxiety more intense than the one I'd experienced after the accident, I screamed, "Get it off! Get it the hell off me!" I tried to throw it off by shaking my head, but I couldn't move. The full body brace had me paralyzed, just the way I'd felt under the truck when a combination of the physical shock and the bag had prevented me from moving.

"We didn't want you to get wet." The paramedics sounded surprised at my violent reaction to their thoughtfulness.

If being blasted with hot air and noise from a running pickup engine five inches above my head had been frightening, lying under the gushing wind and deafening whir of helicopter propellers was finally—and perhaps surprisingly—more than I could bear. Fear, not blood, pulsed through my body.

Although I was starting to hyperventilate, I managed to raise my voice to say, "I can't go in that—take the Long Island Expressway."

Probably aware that I was on the verge of a full-blown panic attack, the EMT barked, "You *are* going—it is protocol for all head injuries to go by air to Stony Brook. I've flown this trip hundreds of times. It'll be okay."

Maybe it was the toughness in the voice of the EMT—who, Ed later told me, looked like an ex-Marine—or maybe it was the forty-five-year-old images of helicopters hovering over jungle clearings stored in my brain, but I was suddenly embarrassed at my cowardice. If soldiers with their legs blown off could be thrust into helicopters under fire from the Viet Cong, I could be lifted gently by friendly EMTs under the watchful eye of my loving husband into a helicopter idling on Wall Street's playground.

I yelled over the helicopter noise, "Okay, I'm on a mission. I'm wounded. You're rescuing me from the Viet Cong. Get me up there. Let's go."

I couldn't see his face, but I imagine the EMT was rolling his eyes. They hoisted the stretcher up and I lay on the helicopter floor, the pilot at my feet and the EMT at my head.

But we didn't take off. The EMT shouted over the noise that if the storm didn't stop in thirty minutes, we'd drive. Then, thirty minutes later, as the rain still fell, he assured me that we could simply fly above it.

If I was going to die in a helicopter crash after being hit by a truck, I thought, so be it. Who was I to interfere with that cosmic plan? I lay in what felt like suspended animation, too tired to revisit my life.

I was sure the EMT meant well as he narrated the trip— "There's Wading River out there. Riverhead's right below us. Wow, there's the racetrack. Did you ever go? We'll be in Stony Brook soon"—but I couldn't stand his chatter. I didn't want to be oriented. I didn't want to be there at all.

The noise suddenly got louder, and two minutes later I was moving very quickly, probably being wheeled on a gurney.

When we stopped just inside the hall at the entrance of the Stony Brook emergency ward, a doctor asked if I was the one from East Hampton.

"Yes," I said, "this is how all the celebrities from East Hampton come to Stony Brook."

Expecting at least a smile from her, I reddened at her wince.

She must have thought that if I was capable of making such a bad joke I was not in danger of dying any time soon. Triage assessment apparently concluded, she left me parked where she found me in the public area outside the emergency room.

Lying flat on my back, I couldn't see anything except the fluorescent lights on the white ceiling above me—so when Ed walked up the hall a few minutes later, I didn't see him approaching. He just suddenly appeared, like at the airport. God knows how fast he drove what was usually an hour-and-a-half trip, and I'd never ask. He smiled down at me, and although I could see that the ends of his mouth were tensed and his forehead was slightly creased, my shoulders relaxed inside the brace.

———

I thought an hour had elapsed between arriving and receiving morphine, but Ed told me later it had been more like three and described the sequence. When he arrived, nurses were huddled around the gurney, asking questions I tried to answer. Apparently, I was distraught and in pain and every time they tried to roll me over to move me onto a hospital bed, I said I was going to throw up and was too dizzy. They tried a few more times and then gave up and left us there in the entrance to the emergency room. I was in some kind of daze, and when a gunshot victim was rushed by us, a flurry of cops trailing his gurney, it didn't even register.

Eventually, I was wheeled into a narrow private room. Unlike a hospital's usual fluorescent glare, the same harsh blue light that sickens me in shopping malls, the only light in this room came from the hall and the red lights flickering on a wall panel. Perhaps they'd kept it dark because of my concussion.

For the first time since I'd entered the hospital, I began to feel a sustained pain shooting through my head, along with an overpowering wave of nausea that started at my feet and gained power as it gushed up to my throat any time I was moved even the slightest bit. I begged the nurse for a painkiller.

"Sorry," she told me, "we can't give you anything until we figure out if you have a brain injury."

"Oh my God. It hurts so much. Who cares about a brain injury? I can't take it. I can't lie here like this anymore."

Ed said something to her, but I was moaning too loud to

hear. At some point, she came back in and said she could give me some Tylenol.

"Are you kidding? Please, it hurts so much. Tylenol is worthless." I might have been whining as much as crying.

"Do you want the Tylenol or not? That's all I can give you until we finish the tests. I can give it to you in a pill or a dropper."

I looked over at Ed. "I can't do a pill. It's going to be too hard. I can't lift my head."

"Okay, dropper then," the nurse said.

I flashed back on those times I'd practically wrestled Peter to the ground when he was a toddler so I could get a dropper into his mouth—amoxicillin, probably. Now, my turn, my karma.

The nurse had to wrestle with me as well. She leaned over and jimmied her arm beneath my shoulders. The second she began to lift, the entire room started spinning and I screamed—out of fear as much as discomfort. She laid me back down.

"Ya know, if you don't let me do this, I just can't do it, and you won't have any medication," she said, a trace of nasal-New-York-wise-guy in her voice.

Jesus, how mean could she be? I don't know what Ed was doing. I guess there wasn't much he could have done. (Luckily, whatever skills he lacked in patient advocacy, he would later make up for in tender patient care.)

"Okay, okay, I want it."

She lifted me with one arm, and I could see the dropper filled with red liquid. I had been picturing a child-size dropper. This one was big enough for a cow. When she squirted it into the side of my mouth just the way I'd seen our veterinarian do to our dog, I smiled to myself.

The motion of easing my head back to the pillow was too

much for me. I threw up, and a projectile of red goop splattered all over the white sheets.

I was embarrassed—not only because what I'd just done was disgusting but also because for a flash I'd allowed myself to feel vindicated, satisfied, victorious for vomiting. This must be how Peter had felt as a toddler: unable to win verbal battles, only able to communicate his disgust by throwing up. For me, it had been easier than telling this nurse what I thought of her bedside manner. But of course, it also scared me. Now I had no hope of any immediate pain relief.

———

Eventually, I was taken to a bright room for tests, where the MRI and X-ray machines seemed to rotate around me. As she wheeled me out, the nurse told me that my test results were good. No broken bones. No internal injuries. I could have some morphine.

I was lying in the hall again, but this time near a nurses' station. Ed was standing to my right. I was still flat on my back. The morphine hadn't done much for the dizziness, but it seemed to have cleared my thinking.

"Did you call Matt?" I asked Ed.

"He knows where you are. He was home with me when the police called. And I called him on my way to Stony Brook."

"Yeah, but he doesn't know what's going on. Call him and tell him I'm okay." Somehow I remembered Peter was in New York City for a few days. No point in worrying him now.

"Look," Ed said, "my cell doesn't get any reception here. I'm going to have to call from outside, and I don't want to lose you.

They might move you somewhere. It took me long enough to find you in the first place."

"Please, I want you to call Matt. And, also, did you tell the Johnsons we're not coming for dinner?"

———

There was no danger of "losing" me, it turned out. I started to regain my sense of time then, so I know for a fact I lay in that hall for hours. Every so often, a doctor came by and raised me ten degrees to see if I threw up. Or chatted with me. One asked, "You're the one from East Hampton who got hit by a truck? I thought it was a little girl."

"But I'm only fifty-seven," I squeaked in my best four-year-old voice.

He shook his head and walked away.

———

Just two weeks earlier, on a friend's recommendation, I had picked up *Change Your Brain, Change Your Life: The Break-through Program for Conquering Anxiety, Depression, Obsessive-ness, Anger, and Impulsiveness*. I'd read the section on how to cope with "cycling" thoughts, the endless loop of worries that plagued me, and it was actually very illuminating, but after a week or so I'd come to the same disappointing conclusion I had reached after doing the visualizations, activities, and prescriptions contained in all the other self-help books lining my shelves: spiritual and emotional transformation was not going to happen for me. Perhaps it was my lack of discipline or patience. I didn't think it was my cognitive ability; after all, I'd had to do some heavy thinking in law school.

But as I lay in the hall of the hospital emergency room, I wondered if it was simply that I, like my seventh-grade students, had required a more immediate, more direct (dare I say concrete?) approach. All I had needed to change my life was to smash my brain on the pavement and wake up in the presence of monks.

I wondered if I was hallucinating, but Ed saw them too. First one and then, after five minutes, another, and soon after that, two by two, a steady stream of Buddhist monks in saffron-colored robes, from young boys to old men, silently walked back and forth past my gurney, on their way to and from the room of a dying monk. I felt overwhelmed by love.

―――

Around midnight, eight hours after the EMTs had brought me in, Doctor Marshall asked if I'd mind having a medical student stitch up my head. I said no.

The doctor and her student discussed the jagged edges of the wound and the angles of the stitches. The first stitch felt like nothing more than a little pinch, but then the doctor handed the needle to the student. "Your turn."

First, some tugging; then, some yanking.

"See how the stitch missed that edge? Let's try that one again."

When for the fourth time Dr. Marshall instructed the student to remove the stitch and try again, I tried to focus on her patience and calm. Perhaps this was a lesson meant for me as well. Hopefully the student learned more from her than I did, because by the eighth do-over I was on the verge of screaming, "What the hell, didn't you learn anything in medical school?"

I kept quiet, but at follow-up appointments when doctors asked how many sutures I'd had, I answered: "Attempted or completed?"

———

I expected to spend at least one night in the hospital, so I was surprised when, about ten hours after the accident, the nurse said that I'd be going home if I could walk. She helped me stand up and I slowly put one foot in front of the other, clutching the side of the bed. I crept a few steps, and then she instructed me to turn around and go back.

"Great job," she said. "After we give you discharge instructions, you can go home."

"Wait, home? In this condition?" I sat back down on the bed and looked over at Ed, slightly shrugging my shoulders.

"I can't believe it either," he said, "but I guess if they say you can go, you can go."

I looked down at my hospital gown, its faint blue stripes blending into a background that, once a crisp hospital white, now matched the gray walls of the room. I wondered how I was going to get dressed.

When I looked up, Ed was holding my black cotton shift. "Can you reach your hands up over your shoulders? I'll slip it over your head."

I looked up at him. "Ed?" I didn't have to add what I was thinking: *Are you kidding? My shoulders and back are killing me.*

"Oh, yeah, right. Sorry."

He gently guided my head through the neck opening and stretched the armholes wide so I could slip my arms through without too much contortion. "Now for the sandals."

Like a child, I lifted my feet straight out in front of me. "What's that on my right foot, on the outside?" There were two parallel black smudges, one about four inches long, the other shorter.

"Oh . . . um . . . I think that's a tire mark."

"What? From the truck?" My breath quickened.

"Yeah, the cop told me at the airport. He was saying how lucky you were. Apparently when the truck was dragging you, it knocked off your sandals, and your foot must have been next to the tire the whole time."

"Oh God." *One more inch and the tire would have run over my foot, my leg, me?* I closed my eyes. "Okay, put on my sandals."

———

An hour later, at 1:30 a.m., I was hurtling home on the LIE, grateful not to be in a helicopter. I stared ahead, unable to process the cars speeding by on my left and right. What would they have felt like rolling over my skin? You expected cars to stay in their lanes—and these vehicles were obeying that simple rule—but then in a second you were on the pavement. Which was weirder: being knocked down by a truck in a crosswalk or going home eleven hours after being knocked down by a truck in a crosswalk?

As I finally lay in my own bed in my own home late that night, surrounded by the comfortingly familiar—the print of the couple lying cheek to cheek under a royal-blue blanket that I'd bought at the Met for my first apartment; the terraced stack of books on my bedside table, my now coverless paperback, *Ayurveda: The Science of Self-Healing,* peeking out from under the bright yellow jacket of *The Lacuna*; our well-worn light blue sheets; my strewn-about bathing suit, shorts, and T-shirts—I was the stranger. Could it really be me lying there, too dizzy to move, my head throbbing, my limbs buzzing? How was I the one with a stiff back and a mind trying to make sense of looking into a rapidly nearing windshield?

I didn't recognize myself.

2

———

WORRYING

AS A CHILD, I LOVED OUR FAMILY'S HOUSE AT 35 VALLEY
Road: its turret whose roof resembled a Chinese peasant's hat;
the attic room, the site of my sister and her friends' "I Hate Boys
Club," whose seven half windows offered a perfect place to look
out for said boys; my bedroom's fireplace, which I longed for
Santa to use one Christmas Eve; the sunlit playroom, whose
large windows created the impression you were playing outside;
and the breakfast room's small, cast-iron potbelly stove, which,
dating back to the house's construction in 1896, was a perpetual
reminder that other children had lived there as well. But despite
our house's considerable size, its playful character was often
overshadowed by my parents' emotional states. The vibrations
of my mother's anger and the damp of my father's depressions
could permeate its every corner and consume me as well. Although I didn't hold the house responsible, at times I would
sense its hidden dangers, those invisible trapdoors through
which my parents might suddenly, at any time, disappear.

Returning home after school during my elementary school
years, I would always run up our front steps, which started from
Valley Road. Those first steps were cut into a three-foot-high
stone retaining wall. To the left was a pink azalea bush that was
taller than me for at least my first seven years. At the top of the

five steps, the stone path, inclining gently, curved to the right to skirt the granite slab, out of the crags of which grew a column of two white and two red azaleas. How reassuring it was that these bushes bloomed each year, ever larger, ever more confident and proud, their power to delight undiminished by the tension within our house. I would run until I reached the cement step that formed the base of the wooden porch staircase, but I never quite gained enough momentum to take those steeply angled steps two by two and always ended up stumbling onto the porch. By the time I reached our front door, a heavy wood Dutch whose top half often remained open to let in the breeze, I would be out of breath.

My anxiety—or "worrying," as it was described back then for children—began with my earliest memories. As a five-year-old, in 1958, I saw my father standing on a balcony at Bronxville's Lawrence Hospital. I didn't know it at the time, but I believe this was about nine months after he'd climbed onto the hotel ledge in New Haven. He had since been moved from a psychiatric facility to Lawrence Hospital, the last stop before returning home.

On the short drive from our house to Lawrence Hospital, Harold and I—four and five years old, born too early for car seats and too excited to sit—stood in the back clutching the front seat to steady ourselves. We drove down the yellow brick hill past the Finleys' home, the site of two childhood amusements. The first was housed in their garage where Mr. Finley kept the '29 red-and-black Duesenberg that he drove, dressed as Santa, to our affluent neighborhood's Christmas parties. The second was McElmoyle, a bulky golden retriever whose escapades delighted us neighborhood kids.

At the bottom of the hill, the road curved around the base of

Sunset Hill, maybe the highest point in Bronxville, site of the Gramatan Hotel, a grand Spanish mission–style building described in the Westchester Archives on Bronxville as the "epitome of high style and elegance" when built in 1905. To me it had always looked like an enchanted castle, and as the hill had once been important to the local Native Americans—where Chief Gramatan might've once watched not only the sunset but also the encroaching white settlers—perhaps it did contain some magic.

When the road wound again, the hospital came into view for just a second but then suddenly disappeared behind stale gray metal and then black shadows as the road sharply dipped under a railroad pass. Years later, I would recognize the railroad bridge for the anomaly that it was in this village of wealthy white Protestant suburbanites who were dedicated to maintaining the manicured landscape and the collective fiction that their lives were as perfect as they appeared to be in the family pictures on their engraved Christmas cards.

Halfway under the bridge and in its darkest shadow, the road rose abruptly. If moving too fast, a car would practically bounce. As we passed under the bridge that day, it could have been the rise in the road or a gravity-defying joy, but I felt like I was flying: the hospital was in view again, and that meant I would see my father for the first time in nine months.

We entered the traffic circle in front of the building, and instead of going left to the entrance and parking lot, we veered off to the right and parked opposite the hospital. (If my mother explained that the hospital prohibited visits by young children, I don't remember.)

My mother rolled down her window and pointed. "Look, look up there, there's Daddy."

We craned our necks. He was standing on a small terrace, about fifty feet up. He was holding the balcony railing with one hand and waving at us, two blond specks inside a dark gray sedan, with the other. Later, looking back, I'd wonder if it had felt strange to him to once again be staring at a sidewalk below.

The best chance Harold and I had to see and be seen was to try to squeeze our heads and arms out of the car window, but the opening was too small for both of us. It was a situation that ordinarily we would have settled by clawing each other until one of us surrendered. However, the visit was too important to waste a minute of it fighting or risk having it cut short as punishment, so we instead engaged in something that might have resembled a mythical dance—first four arms flailing, then two heads bobbing, then any combination thereof, like some frantic blond Shiva. "There's Daddy, there's Daddy!" we shouted.

I don't remember whether Louise and Jimmy were also in the car. At two, Jim may have been too young to come; at ten, Louise may have been sitting in the front with our mother, far enough to be out of reach of the backseat fray.

Although I could hardly have read my brother's thoughts, we must have shared the same magical belief—that if we just yelled louder or waved more wildly, our father would swoop down from the balcony, envelop us in a hug, and come home.

After a few minutes of yelling out to him, I must have realized that he was not going to swoop down, let alone come home, because I felt the mudslide beginning: a thick and heavy sadness that filled every crevice, burying every hiding place, any last refuge for joy. My mother pulled the car out of its parking place.

If the car bounced as we passed back under the bridge, I couldn't feel it.

Although I didn't recognize it until much later, that visit gave rise not only to my first clear memory of my father but also to the unshakable certainty that, at least in our family, happiness should always carry its own kind of weight, its own counterbalance of sadness.

———

In another early memory of my father, he abruptly pushed me off his knee as we sat in the barn-red wicker rocking chair on the front porch. I believe this incident occurred on a short visit home during the year he spent in the hospital after the ledge incident, though I'm not certain that home visits were allowed. As a child, I conflated the push with his absence and decided he'd been away to have his knee fixed. I doubt I knew the word "surgery" or "operation" at that age, but I must have intuited that this explanation was far less scary than the truth, which I wouldn't learn about until I was sixteen.

But even the truth would turn out to be less devastating than the realization I had on the porch that day—that after suddenly abandoning us, our father could return and just as suddenly stop loving us.

———

I worried in elementary school: forgetting my homework, a routine occurrence for other eight-year-olds, would reduce me to sobs. Admitting that I'd lost the Halloween money I'd collected, probably no more than three dollars, felt like a crime of the utmost moral failing.

My favorite teacher, Dr. Berkness, a tall and soft woman in her fifties, had ways to soothe me. On a particularly bad day, she would ask me to walk beside her as the rest of the class tried to patter along single file down the hall. She would squeeze my hand three times, slowly and deliberately, so that there could be no misinterpretation. Our secret code: I-Love-You. As I squeezed back, I could have melted into her arms.

Dr. Berkness's empathy permeated her classroom even in the form of the wall hangings. I loved sitting under the protective gaze of the grid of multiplication tables, whose bold black numbers remained the same each day. As Dr. Berkness wrote in my third-grade report, "Amy seems to carry the weight of the world on her shoulders. As I mentioned at parent conferences, I am trying to do something about that."

Fifth grade was worse because I had a teacher, a man for the first time, who smiled but whose black, shiny hair and equally dark mustache reminded me of someone who didn't have any feelings: a gangster or an accountant, maybe.

It didn't help when one day the school psychologist—who everyone knew spent time with "kids with problems"—appeared in the door of our classroom and my teacher, after walking over to her and leaning down so she could whisper in his ear, then announced to the class: "Amy, go with Dr. Beisel."

I knew already that something must be wrong with me, and staring at the series of black blobs printed on white cards didn't reassure me.

"Okay, Amy, now just tell me what that reminds you of."

I picked a word that I thought a girl with nothing wrong with her would say: "Dog."

"And this one?"

"Dog."

"Okay, Amy, what about this picture?"

"Umm, like a dog, I think."

"Really? You're sure about that?"

"Yes, pretty sure: a dog."

No one ever told me why I'd been sent to the school psychologist. But as far as I could tell, nothing changed after that visit. I continued to worry.

———

That's not to say I didn't love school. After all, my parents prized books and education above all else, so reading, learning, and exploring had become a way for me to stay connected to them.

If that connection came with anxiety, so be it.

In fifth grade, I started learning to play the clarinet. Twice a week, I would walk with another girl in my class to Mr. Mingrone's music room in the junior high school wing. About ten fifth and sixth graders sat in semicircular rows, holding silver-keyed black horns between our legs, tensing our lips around the reeds and waiting for the signal to blow. My right hand was reliable: as each finger lifted, the sound was low, steady, and soothing. But as soon as I proceeded to the higher notes, my left-hand ring finger would release a series of squeaks as embarrassing and unpredictable as an adolescent boy's changing voice. Many of the other kids were squeaking too, but their mistakes sounded ordinary and forgivable. To me, mine announced a congenital unworthiness.

I suppose a little extra practice might have taken care of the problem, but that didn't occur to me. I dreaded clarinet lessons and eventually began to complain loudly of headaches, stomach pains, sore throats, and, if the timing was right, burning fevers (which I faked by holding the thermometer against the light bulb for a minute, a trick I'd learned from TV) on Tuesday and Thursday mornings. When my mother, with Mr. Mingrone's help, discovered the pattern in my ailments, she insisted I go to school.

"No, I can't," I insisted. "I can't go today. I feel terrible. My stomach hurts. I think I'm going to throw up."

"Amy, there is absolutely nothing wrong with your stomach. I talked to Mr. Mingrone, and I know you have lessons today. You can't stay home. He says you're one of his best students." My mother's glare was already fixed—no chance for any sympathy to sneak in—but I couldn't give up.

"I am *not* one of the best. I'm not as good as Louise Fletcher. He just doesn't want kids to quit."

"Amy, *get dressed.*"

"If you make me go, I'm going to"—I wasn't sure I could say it, but I was not going to sit in that band room again—"kill myself."

"You have to go to school, and that's it!"

If she'd taken me seriously or thought about my father's attempt, I think there would have been a trace of concern in her facial expression or voice. But I don't blame her for her insensitivity—or maybe I've since forgiven her. And perhaps my outburst was just the ordinary and stubborn refusal of a privileged, suburban ten-year-old. But as I turned away from her and screamed those words, it truly felt like a matter of life and death. I couldn't stand sitting in that band room, continuously reminded that no matter how hard I tried not to, I would keep making mistakes.

And through my mother's constant warnings at home, I'd

learned that making mistakes could have serious consequences. If I told her about a problem with a friend or with schoolwork, she would look me in the eye and say, "Don't tell Dad about that; it might get him upset" (or "mad" or "worried"). Or, if my brothers and I were getting rambunctious, she would tell us (probably more accurately, yell at us) to "quiet down," "go somewhere else," or "stop running" so we didn't "bother Dad." On the few occasions when I asked her why, she paused, made sure to look me in the eye, and said, "Dad's sick, Amy." So I closely monitored my behavior around him, but I still worried that, out of carelessness or ignorance, I might say or do the wrong thing. And making a mistake that would upset Dad felt like a deadly gamble.

One night during the clarinet battle, I snuck a plastic dry-cleaning bag under the covers of my bed. Its warning about suffocation had given me the idea. I lay there in the dark holding the bag over my head and face, hoping someone would discover my misery. I squeezed the bottom around my neck until I couldn't stand the pounding pressure in my head and the burning in my face.

I can't say this was a suicide attempt; it was, perhaps, more like a test to find out whether my parents would save me. But I knew they were unlikely to come to my room after bedtime unless I yelled for them, and that would defeat the purpose. My test, in the end, was half-hearted. Perhaps even then I sensed the truth: They weren't capable of saving me. They were too busy trying to save themselves.

I went to clarinet a few more times before I eventually won the battle. My mother's interpretation, which she shared with Mr. Mingrone and anyone else interested, was that I had sensitive ears and couldn't stand all the squeaking.

———

I didn't know why my father was sick, and it didn't occur to me to ask. My mother, it seemed to me, couldn't be interrupted. As she used to say with equal measures of pride and exasperation, she had "three under three": my brother, Harold, born thirteen months after me, and then Jimmy, who arrived seventeen months after Harold. My mother's strength was obvious. As she stomped around the house, always on a mission, a rush of air rivaling a humpback's exhale would force its way through her perennially clenched jaw and pursed lips every five minutes or so. For her, even the need to breathe seemed to be an admission of weakness. She needed every bit of that power to maintain her grip on the cliff edge from which she was dangling. Let up for a second and she would pick up a drink.

Much later, she told me that during her years as an active alcoholic, she'd been a "periodic." She could stop drinking for a month or so, but then once she started up again she couldn't stop until she'd hit a bottom of sorts. I imagine one of those times might have been when she was pulled over while driving home around 1:00 a.m. after a night of drinking.

Apparently, the village cop who pulled her over on one of Bronxville's many quiet suburban streets was very polite.

"Mrs. Turner, you were swerving back there." In the one-square-mile village of Bronxville, the police knew most residents by name.

"Yes, officer, I was, and I don't care," my mother responded.

"Ma'am, have you been drinking tonight?"

"Yes, I've 'been drinking tonight.'" She mimicked his official tone. And then, slurring, she added, "So whaaaat."

"You're going to have to get out of the car, Mrs. Turner," he said, his tone still patient and polite. After all, this was the fifties in an all-white, affluent suburb of New York City.

"And then," she told me when she recounted this story to me years later, when I was in my twenties—and she reddened as she spoke—"I got out of the car and walked over to the sidewalk. I was shaky, clearly a little wobbly. I leaned against the hood of my car on the sidewalk side. He told me to wait there and walked back around to the driver's side of his car. But just as he was rounding the rear of his car, I ran over to the passenger window, reached through, grabbed the microphone attached to the car megaphone, and shouted as loud as I could, 'I AM VIRGINIA TURNER AND I'M DRUNK AS HELL AND I DON'T CARE WHO KNOWS IT!'"

"Jesus, Mom, really?" I asked. My face was probably as flushed as my mother's. Knowing how much she loathed excessive displays of emotion, it never occurred to me that her drinking problem would have been so public.

She shook her head with a half chuckle. "Yep, really. I don't even know if I got a ticket. But I do know a lot of people heard me that night."

She stopped drinking about a month after my father went into the hospital.

From an early age, I knew she went to meetings. I must have been about eight when she came home one night around 9:00 p.m. I heard her in the kitchen and ran down to greet her. "Mom, Mrs. Bennett called."

"Oh, thanks. What did she say?"

"Um, I have it here." I looked down at my handwriting, which I'd carefully copied over in pen. I was proud of this scrap, my first real phone message. "She said to call her tomorrow."

"Thank you, Amy. Good job. What did you tell her?"

"I said you were at a meeting." I recalled the feeling of pride as I told Mrs. Bennett where she was. In my estimation, only important people went to meetings.

"Amy." She glared slightly. "Don't ever tell anyone I'm at a meeting."

————

A few years later, my mother looked over at me in the passenger seat in the midst of us running errands together and announced that she had to stop by someone's house to talk to her. "Someone who is having trouble with their drinking."

We parked in the lot of one of the very few apartment buildings in Bronxville. It was a novelty for me to ride in an elevator.

My mother knocked, and a woman opened the door. Her brown hair was scraggly, and she was wearing a housecoat. She didn't seem to notice me; she just looked directly at my mother and said, "Thanks, Virginia," then turned away from us and walked back through the hall to the kitchen.

We followed. She stood at the sink and turned on the faucet. In the window in front of her, a few green leaves fluttered against the blue sky. I was scared.

"Joyce, what's going on?" My mother's voice sounded tough. Nothing like what I expected when you tried to help someone in trouble. "Answer me: When did you start drinking?"

The woman started to whimper.

"Joyce?"

The woman started crying. I was embarrassed for her. I

knew I shouldn't be there. This was for grown-ups, I thought, private. I didn't even understand what was happening. Why would my mother bring me here? I sat on the floor and bent forward to stare at my feet, hoping I might disappear if I could curl up small enough.

They sat next to each other on the couch. My mother talked sternly; the woman cried quietly and nodded, pausing occasionally to utter a "yeah," "okay," or "uh-huh." I was also embarrassed by my mother. Her tone was so gruff. And this woman was *crying*. How could she be so mean? Why wasn't she soothing her the way you're supposed to when someone is in pain?

When I heard the woman's intermittent sobs relax into sniffles, I looked up and was surprised to see her smiling gingerly at my mother and repeating, "Thank you so much, Virginia. Thank you, really."

"Okay, Joyce. I'll be back at six thirty. The meeting's at seven. Don't drink too much." My mother smiled wryly.

The woman laughed.

I would learn later that the visit was, in AA parlance, a "twelve-step" call. And as I learned more about AA, I understood that what I'd thought was gruffness and meanness in my mother's tone had simply been directness and honesty. A sober alcoholic talking to an active alcoholic. No room for mincing words, no quarter for denial. But I still don't understand why I accompanied her. I prefer to think that it was an emergency and she'd had no alternative. Otherwise, I might have to consider that she was too unaware or preoccupied to even consider the visit's impact on me.

During those years, I worried about my father for reasons I didn't yet fully understand. But I also worried for reasons I couldn't ignore. Unlike the reasons for his yearlong hospitalization, my father's political activism—which generated substantial controversy in our village and publicity elsewhere—was no secret in our family. Apparently, his hospitalization had effected a dramatic change: it had propelled him into a lifelong mission to fight injustice, perhaps to save himself as much as others. Until then, he had not been involved in political or social issues. He might have been considered a conservative (at least anti-FDR) in college, and an apathetic Republican thereafter. But about two years after his release from the hospital, he co-wrote a letter to the local paper challenging Bronxville's longstanding exclusion of people because of their "race or religion," a practice that was never discussed publicly but was obvious in the exclusively white and majority Protestant population of that square mile.

About four years later, in early 1965, my father would help form the "Concerned Citizens of Bronxville," a committee that initially consisted only of my parents and one other couple whose mission was to support the local hospital's predominantly Black workers in their efforts to join Hospital Workers Union 1199—a situation my father became aware of through conversations with our housekeeper, Doretha, whose husband, Matt, was a hospital orderly. That two-year effort would involve marches down the main street, noisy picketing on the sidewalks outside the hospital, and the use of billy clubs by the village's police, which drew comparisons, unwanted even in Bronxville, to what was happening at the time to demonstrators in Selma, Alabama.

During this period, some of my classmates became suddenly uncomfortable around me, looking down or away as I passed by.

A few others confronted me with snippets of conversations they must have heard at home. Richard—blond like me, slightly chubby, and generally menacing only when he was standing behind the class bully—walked up as I waited my turn to play tetherball.

"You know, your parents are killing people," he said.

"What?" I stumbled back a few steps, as much out of shock as a desire to escape. "What do you mean?"

"There's nobody working in the hospital. They're all marching outside. My mother says patients are gonna"—he jutted out his chin for emphasis—"*die* in there if they don't stop."

I had nothing to say. I thought it might be true. And my parents *were* picketing with them. I squeezed my mouth shut, hoping the force might stop the tears beginning to blur my vision.

Sensing drama, the tetherball players stopped; other twelve-year-olds gathered in a semicircle behind Richard.

My best friend, Loren, stepped forward. It helped that she was about six inches taller than my accuser.

"My grandmother's in that hospital," she said. "And she likes it. She says the songs those marchers sing are really nice." In a nasal tone suggesting the childish taunt "nyah, nyah," she added, jutting *her* chin forward, "Cheers her up."

My classmates didn't seem persuaded, but they drifted away when it was clear Richard had no comeback.

Although I felt a rush of gratitude for Loren's intervention, I could no longer ignore that our family had become a sort of collective pariah. Of course, my parents' involvement in the strike was worse for my older sister, who faced more articulate attacks from her high school classmates. And although she claimed that it was a badge of honor not to be selected to "come out" at the local cotillion, the exclusion must have hurt.

As press coverage expanded to the *New York Times*—"Police and Pickets Clash at Hospital; 26 Seized and 2 Hurt"—Bronxville's residents were getting angrier. My mother joined my father in most of his activities. She had no personal need to be a martyr, but she had a strong sense of fairness and of course would not want to risk jeopardizing their marriage or her husband's emotional stability by refusing to help. But it wasn't easy on her. Although a column about her and another woman in the *New York Post* titled "The Valiant" must have been encouraging, she lost a lot of so-called friends and began to receive a frosty reception, at best, at the local club where she loved to play tennis.

One afternoon, after she picked me up from school, my mother and I walked into one of the two drugstores that bookended Bronxville's main street. I was hoping she'd buy me an ice cream soda.

Steinmann's plate glass windows and high ceilings made its large interior light and airy, too open for a customer to avoid detection. We were no more than five steps into the drugstore when a man sitting on a red leather–cushioned counter stool twirled around to face us. His shout was so loud it seemed to echo off the gleaming surfaces.

"Goddamn it, there she is. There's that goddamn n— lover. Why don't you get the hell out? GET THE HELL OUT."

My mother froze for the second it took to gasp, then grabbed my hand and yanked me toward the door. As we pushed against its heavy glass, I could still hear the man's shouts and then, perhaps just a little too late, the owner's voice saying, "I'm sorry, Mrs. Turner. I'm sorry."

Sitting in the front seat of the car, I was too scared to speak. The image of the man's face, red and crinkled with rage, would not recede; his knobby finger jabbing at the air still felt like punctures. My mother looked over at me, then down at the seat, then closed her eyes and shook her head slowly.

A few words from her might have been reassuring, but I don't know what she could have said. Her look was more comforting: sheer hatred could pierce adults as well. We sat there for a few moments in silence before she drove us home.

———

Although my parents must have tried to hide what they could, I knew they'd received telephoned death threats and hate mail. And none of us could miss the police cars circling our house during a party my parents gave for the Black hospital workers and Jewish union organizers—a perceived threat, even if they were in Bronxville only for a social visit.

I couldn't risk "getting Dad upset" by telling him that I wanted him to stop, wanted people to like us again, wanted my friends back. He was selfish, I thought. It wasn't fair. I had already been worrying about him because of his "illness," but that, I sensed, was beyond his control. Now, by supporting the strike, he was causing me additional worry on purpose and didn't seem to care. I wanted to return to the normal amount of worrying.

I did take some comfort, warranted or not, in the expression of support from a stranger. After school one afternoon, I had just run up the path by the bare azalea bushes and bounded through the front door at 35 Valley when I heard my mother shout, "Amy, look what came today! It's on the front table." There was a

half sheet of yellow tissue paper stamped MARCH 31, 1965, 2:37
P.M.:

I HAD HOPED TO PHONE YOU WHILE IN THIS CITY, BUT
PRESSURE OF ACTIVITIES COMPELS ME TO LEAVE FOR
BALTIMORE. THEREFORE I EXTEND MY PERSONAL
CONGRATULATIONS FOR YOUR INVALUABLE
CONTRIBUTION IN ASSURING SUCCESSFUL OUTCOME OF
BRONXVILLE HOSPITAL STRIKE. EFFECTIVE UNITY OF
LOCAL 1199, CIVIL RIGHTS MOVEMENT, AND YOUR
CONCERNED CITIZENS COMMITTEE HAS BLAZED A
TRAIL FOR ALL OF LABOR TO EMULATE. I JOIN WITH MY
FELLOW FREEDOM FIGHTERS IN THE SOUTH IN
SALUTING YOUR COURAGE IN ACHIEVING AN
IMPORTANT VICTORY IN OUR COMMON STRUGGLE FOR
HUMAN AND UNION RIGHTS.

DR. MARTIN LUTHER KING JR.

She didn't have to explain to me who Martin Luther King Jr.
was. He and the civil rights movement were a frequent topic of
conversation around the house. And two years earlier, my father
had attended the August March on Washington, which the rest
of our family had tried to watch at our summer house in Wainscott on the snowy screen of our TV.

Although the telegram removed any lingering doubt about
the justness of my parents' cause, it also made me more ashamed
of my selfishness. Dr. King's approval made it indisputable that
my father had done the right thing, taken a courageous stand. I
was very proud of him. Proud of all of us. And yet I still wanted
him to stop, to put my needs first.

To admire my father for the same reason I resented him was confusing and uncomfortable. I was not yet ready to accept the adult reality of yin-yang feelings, that opposing feelings could be equally justified and accepted as essential parts of the whole.

And the telegram couldn't quite eradicate my hurt and disappointment, the source of which I didn't yet fully recognize, that the strength my father demonstrated in the strike did not enable him to handle his own emotional problems, or those of his children.

3

LOOKING FOR NORMAL

EIGHTEEN HOURS AFTER MY COLLISION WITH THE TRUCK, I lay in bed at home, noticing how the dust diffused the light hitting the window at the end of the hall. That was about all the stimulation I could process. I was waiting and, once again, on guard.

I scanned my body for signs: Where was I on this supposed road to recovery? Was this the worst I would feel? Would the next weeks bring a gradual easing of the throbbing in my head, the pinching on my scalp, the stiffness in my joints, and a fatigue so deep it seemed to have displaced my bone marrow? Or was this just the beginning of serious complications like brain damage, loss of language, and weakened limbs? After all, I thought, how do you walk away from getting hit by a truck?

Before he left for work a few hours earlier, Ed had made sure everything I needed was either on the bedside table or his side of the bed: the cordless phone, a glass of water, the *New York Times*, a mug of coffee, and a slice of toast and jam. I was too nauseated to eat, but his gesture was comforting nonetheless.

The sound of footsteps coming up the staircase excited me out of my half sleep. It was Matt. Almost twenty-four and standing at six-two or so, Matt could have easily touched the top of the door. The summer sun had already tipped the balance in his hair color to the light blond of his childhood. The color of his eyes, however, never changed. Midnight blue at the outermost edges, his irises gradually lightened in concentric bands until they framed the pupils in a hint of white. Today they were slightly clouded.

"Hey, Mom, do you want some lunch? I was going to make you something, maybe like a sandwich?"

My upper back softened into the pillows, releasing a tension that I hadn't been aware of. Matt had few domestic skills and had previously showed no interest in acquiring more. He could be helpful, but only when asked. So, although he, like his father, had difficulty expressing his feelings, today his message was clear: he was concerned about me.

When we'd come through the front door at three o'clock that morning, I must have looked strange, if not scary—stooped over and leaning on Ed's arm, a white bandage wrapped around my head, wearing the sleeveless black cotton shift and platform sandals in which I'd left the house twelve hours earlier. Standing in the hall, Matt had hesitated, his eyes crinkling slightly, as though he were assessing whether it was safe to come closer to me. Ed had walked me over to him, and Matt had bent down so I could hug his shoulders.

"Don't worry, I'm alright, really," I'd said before Ed led me upstairs.

Still bandaged, but no doubt appearing less concerning now that I was in bed, I smiled up at Matt. "A sandwich? Oh, thanks so much, sweetie, but I'm not hungry. You don't have to bother with that." I should have let him do it, but I was unwilling to admit I needed help, unwilling even to give my son the opportunity to demonstrate his love. Although Matt seemed unfazed, my disappointment for both of us trailed him down the stairs.

———

A few hours later, my sister, Louise, called.

"Hi, how's it going?" she asked, not yet aware of the accident.

"Oh yeah, thanks. I wanted to tell you about something, but before I do, I just wanted to say I'm sorry for being so intense in our last conversation. I felt bad about it. I was going to call you to apologize, but—"

"About what? I don't remember anything intense."

"You know, that thing about Mom."

"Oh, okay. I hadn't really thought about it."

"Well, good. But anyway, I got hit by a truck yesterday, but I'm okay."

"What? Oh my God, really? I can't believe it." Her voice was getting faster and higher. "Yesterday? And now you're home and okay?"

"Yeah, and it was so ridiculous." I told her the story of carrying my dry cleaning, the truck hitting me head-on. "And I was lying under this truck in the dark, and I was thinking I was going to die suffocating on my dry cleaning!"

"My God, that was serious. It must have been terrifying."

"Yeah, well, a little scary, I guess, but you know, I'm so lucky. I'm not hurt, just a concussion. It could have been so much worse. It's not that bad."

"But Amy," she said, her voice descending an octave or two, "that was an unbelievable trauma."

"No, Louise, really. It wasn't. I'm okay. I mean, I was lying there talking about the teacher's union and that time I brought the squirrel to the dry cleaners. I bet they were all cracking up."

She tried one more time. "I can't believe you're laughing about this. You must have been so scared. I mean, *a truck just mowed you down.*"

She was right, but admitting that made me feel like I was looking into a mirror at a wound oozing across my face or descending into an abyss, a feeling I always associated with my father. *I am not sick*, I repeated to myself.

"I'm *telling* you, it wasn't that big a deal," I cut in. "*I'm okay*—I don't have any broken bones, and I'm basically back to normal. I *don't* want to talk about it anymore. How are things in Sarasota?"

Based on Louise's reaction, I decided after I hung up the phone to notify my brother. Jim's strict sense of boundaries would have prevented him from questioning my glibness, but even so I was grateful that he generally preferred communicating by email. As for Harold . . . although by then he had been sober for three years, we had grown apart during his decades of heavy drinking. I didn't know what to expect from him, and I didn't have the energy to find out.

4

REVELATIONS

THE INVISIBLE TRAPDOORS I'D FEARED SINCE EARLY childhood finally got a name in 1968 when my parents sent me, at fifteen, to Dr. Ferdinand Jones, a psychologist. Unlike my visit to the school psychologist in fifth grade, I had an idea what had prompted my parents to send me to "Dr. Ferdinand," as I called him. A few weeks earlier, they'd come home from a dinner out and discovered me lying on the living room floor smoking a cigarette, Grateful Dead music blasting from the cabinet stereo. In many families, this behavior would be dismissed as that of a typical teenager, but my father believed that any conduct that suggested an emotional problem should be dealt with "professionally."

My mother, I believe, would have initially opposed sending me to a therapist. She smoked two packs a day without worry and at this point saw therapy as the first stop on the family track to the mental hospital. For her, taking action, not struggling with words and lost memories, was the appropriate line of attack. Thus, a few nights after the cigarette-smoking incident, she dumped in the garbage the baggy, unwashed jeans and stretched-out, ribbed navy sweater that I wore almost every day to school.

But her approach failed: I retrieved them from the trash can, and the next day I wore those same clothes to school. Standing in my bedroom doorway that night, she said—pounding each word, a slight hiss escaping through her clenched teeth—"I don't know why you don't have better self-esteem."

Discussion over, she closed my bedroom door with just enough emphasis to suggest a slam. I sat back down on my bed and thought to myself, *I don't either.*

———

Like almost all parenting tasks, the responsibility of driving me to my weekly therapy session with Dr. Ferdinand was my mother's. It couldn't have been easy for her to sit with a sullen teenager for the thirty-minute drive, wait for another forty-five, then drive home listening to me cry.

Dr. Ferdinand was a Sarah Lawrence professor of psychology who resembled Richie Havens. He had a deep and gravelly voice that to me conveyed the comfort and reassurance of a parent's unconditional hug. And of even more importance to a teenager in the sixties like me, Dr. Ferdinand was cool. Along with the papers and books on his desk were always a few album covers, mostly jazz.

It was a relief to talk to someone. I talked mostly about my parents—how my mother was gruff and so mean to my father. I didn't know why she was so impatient with him. He would tell a silly story to make us laugh, and my mother would shake her head and walk away, saying, "Oh, Harold," with a snort. I told him about our family dinners in the dining room, where my parents sat at the ends, far enough away from each other so that my father could pretend he didn't hear my mother muttering under

her breath each time he prolonged dinner with long explanations of topics of interest only to himself or excused himself to
retrieve something he'd forgotten. When he suddenly interrupted
birthday dinners to "go get something," we would eventually
hear the sounds of papers rustling as he hurriedly wrapped a
present for the child whose birthday we were celebrating that
night. Other evenings, he'd leave the dinner table for shorter
periods, his well-worn volumes of Shakespeare or Aeschylus easier to locate and bring back to the table promptly. Then we'd be
treated to some form of edification. I rarely understood what he
was reading out loud to us, but at least it was usually in a language I recognized.

One night, as my father began reading *Beowulf* in Middle
English, I could hear "For God's sake, Harold" rumbling like
distant thunder from my mother's end, but my father continued,
unfazed by his family's lack of interest.

When these family dinners finally drained the last drop of
patience from my mother's admittedly low reservoir, she would
cut him off with an exhale that would have blown out the birthday candles of an octogenarian followed by, "Harold, the children have homework!"—each word spit out in that "I mean
business" tone she used when she had needed to stop three toddlers dead in their tracks.

Although my father could be absentminded and oblivious to
the mundane needs of his captive audience of children, I
couldn't understand why she showed him so little respect; she
would never tolerate anyone treating her that way.

And, more than wanting my parents to treat each other the
way I thought a married couple should, I wanted them to be
"normal" in other ways too. I wanted my father to be like the

other fathers who every morning took the 7:20 to the city and returned on the 5:45. I wanted him to stand on the station platform with his fedora and briefcase and a rolled-up *New York Times* under his arm, chatting with the other men about stocks or the Knicks or whatever else those men talked about. They looked like a row of columns: if slightly stony, definitely capable of handling the stresses of life. And although I knew it was irrational, I blamed the other fathers for not including mine, as though with just their invitation he might be transformed into one of them.

My mother was different too. She rarely wore a dress or makeup unless she was going out. She was five-eight, long-legged, and slim—tennis kept her in shape all year—but I didn't appreciate her athletic ability or that her daily outfit of slacks and sweaters might be ahead of her time. She didn't like to cook or clean or do anything the other mothers in the neighborhood seemed to enjoy. She couldn't understand how they could follow the same routine every week: laundry on Tuesdays, errands on Wednesdays, grocery shopping on Fridays, and so on. "It would drive me crazy," she told me once, exhaling an extra cloud of smoke, which might have been from one of the cigarillos, narrow cigars with plastic filter tips, that she smoked for a time. I confided to Dr. Ferdinand that I was nervous that she was "like a man, the cigars and pants and all."

Perhaps it was just too confusing as I approached the age when I would have to define femininity for myself.

I doubt Dr. Ferdinand told my mother to change her style, but I do know that he advised my parents to hug us, much to the embarrassment of me and my younger brothers. Other than a daily goodnight kiss from my mother and cherished, though occasional, hand-holding with my father, we typically engaged in little other physical contact in my family. But a few months into my therapy, my father started hugging us—or, more accurately, wrapping his arms around us but making sure that our bodies didn't touch. "Gee, Ame," my brother Harold would say, "it's *SO* weird."

Therapy gave me the courage one night to confront my father about how my mother treated him.

"Dad, Mom is so mean to you. How can you stand it?"

"Oh . . . honey," he said, a tender smile forming at the edges of his mouth.

"I mean. She cuts you off and acts like you're so stupid. She's horrible." And then I raised my voice, not caring who heard me, to say, "I *hate* her."

I couldn't believe I'd said it. We were not a family who expressed their feelings, especially such ugly ones. My eyelids burned and I held back tears. I waited for him to admit it, to tell me that he hated her too.

"Oh, Ame, honey. I love Mom."

"How could you?" I sobbed. "She's so mean."

My father, who was sitting on the edge of my bed, patted my shoulder. "I don't think she's mean. I love her, and I hope you do too, sweetie."

I was quiet then, totally in shock. What was all that tension between them about if they loved each other? I understood nothing.

And of course I told Dr. Ferdinand about my mother's directive: "Don't get Dad upset, Dad's sick, Dad can't handle it."

"Do you have any idea why she says that so often?" Dr. Ferdinand asked.

"No, but she gets this look when she says it. Like something really serious will happen if we get him . . . I don't know, just . . . bad." I looked down at my lap. The fold in my navy sweater couldn't disguise the flesh cresting at the waistband of my jeans.

"Have you ever asked her about it?" Dr. Ferdinand's legs remained slightly outstretched, his ankles crossed.

My face reddened. In Dr. Ferdinand's soothing voice, that option sounded so easy—a natural response to curiosity. But if the impulse to question my mother had ever started to percolate, I had squelched it immediately.

"Oh God. I couldn't. *She would freak out.*"

Years later I would wonder if remaining ignorant had also allowed me to imagine my own, less disturbing outcomes of upsetting my father.

———

Dr. Ferdinand began most sessions by asking me about school or the music I was listening to, but on one afternoon, a few months into my therapy, he started right in.

"I spoke to your mother this week."

I dug my jagged thumbnail under the edge of a Jujube-sized freckle on my forearm and instant-replayed the week, trying to think of what I might have done wrong.

"No, Amy, please, nothing to be concerned about. It's not unusual for therapists to talk to parents, especially when they might be able to help somehow."

I pursed my lips. I couldn't imagine my mother helping, *ever*.

"I asked her if she had any idea what might be causing you

to worry so much about your father. She was surprised to hear you were so concerned."

I pictured my mother sitting on the bed in Louise's room, out of earshot of my father, gripping the black handset with one hand and holding a cigarette in the other—her jaw clenched, her lips pressed together as though blotting lipstick. She didn't want to discuss my feelings. *"Dwelling on your emotions is not going to help, Amy. Just do something."*

"She told me something about your father that she hasn't told you or your brothers because she thought it was too upsetting. I assured her it's healthier for people, including teenagers, to know the facts, even if they're unsettling. She agreed that I should tell you—that is, if you want me to . . ."

I flattened my thumb over the freckle to stanch the red gunk oozing at its edges. I palmed the padded leather arms of the chair and straightened out of my slouch. Dr. Ferdinand waited for me to look up.

"When you were about four or so, your father was on a business trip with a colleague, staying in a hotel in New Haven. Your mother said that he'd gotten *extremely depressed* . . ."

I crossed my knees tightly enough to pretzel my right ankle behind my left, hoping I could cut off the heat rushing through me.

"Your father became so distraught, and this might be hard to hear, but he climbed outside his window, out onto the ledge . . ."

My insides hiccupped, as though every organ had all at once gasped. To anchor myself, I stared at Dr. Ferdinand. As the air thickened, his words seemed to trudge toward me.

"A priest talked to him, and your father came back inside.

After that he was hospitalized for about a year, but your mother said he's never done anything like that again."

I looked down and exhaled slowly. As I closed my eyes, brimming tears escaped. The revelation was utterly shocking and strangely familiar; it was as though the family photographs on our annual Christmas cards had suddenly changed, our forced smiles now accompanied by a darkness around the eyes. For the first time, I understood why my mother's warnings had been so serious, why they'd carried a hint of life-and-death consequences, why I'd felt the need to protect him.

"You mean, he was going to jump off the ledge?"

"Well, if he *was* going to do that, remember that he changed his mind."

"Then he went to a hospital . . . like an insane asylum?"

"A psychiatric hospital, we'd call it, where I'm sure he had excellent doctors, received a lot of therapy, medications, treatments . . ."

"Like shock treatments?" I'd read *One Flew Over the Cuckoo's Nest*.

"Well, yes. But it's nothing like you might be picturing, and the hospitalization must have helped, of course."

"Maybe that was the year I thought he was having a knee operation or becoming a doctor . . ."

"I'm sure this is hard on you." Dr. Ferdinand cocked his head, one side of his mouth inched upward. "But with most people, having things out in the open helps. It really does. Now we can talk about it in here, and my hope is that you'll have a lot less worry."

After that session, as I slumped into the passenger seat of our car, my mother quickly folded the *New York Times* she'd been reading and placed it on the floor at my feet. The cigarette that she clenched, FDR-like, held on to its dangling ash.

"Ready to go?" she asked, a little too optimistically. My face, reddened from crying, had taken on the added hue of fury. *Every minute of every day for the past twelve years, I have been living in a parallel universe of my mother's creation, under her total control.* I didn't hold my father accountable for keeping the secret; he was "sick," as I was so often reminded. It would be years before I could appreciate how excruciating my father's ordeal would have been for her, an active alcoholic with four children under the age of nine.

On the drive home, I plotted my revenge: revealing the truth to my brothers, which I knew would infuriate her. (Louise was away at college and would've already known about my father's attempt, as she had been nine at the time of the event.) Born so close together, my brothers and I had been a force from the beginning. We'd vanquished babysitter after babysitter. Live-in housekeepers would escape in the night, presumably ashamed to admit that they were no matches for three towheaded toddlers. That we were preverbal was absolutely no obstacle to our planning and execution. We were invincible. Back then, the three of us were of one indestructible piece: even we couldn't tell where one of us ended and the other began.

Like a teenage Deep Throat, I approached my brothers that afternoon—separately, so as not to arouse my mother's suspicion—and told them, "Seven o'clock, my room. I need to tell you something. And you better not tell Mom, or I will kill you. She'll be at an AA meeting."

Unfortunately, I'd forgotten that the Thursday AA meetings didn't start until seven thirty. And thus just moments after

I had blabbed, my mother walked into my bedroom to see me, sitting on my twin bed, facing Harold and Jimmy on the guest bed opposite me, the three of us crouched so far forward that our knees were touching. Another parent might have thought we were rolling a joint, but my mother knew exactly what was happening, and that she was too late. The shock had already registered on my brothers' faces and in their voices as they had whispered their questions to me in an anxious duet, "What? Wait, what did you say? Are you sure? He was going to jump? You mean he had shock treatments?" And then there had been just enough time for our nervous giggles, the ones that invariably escape whenever teenagers enter unfamiliar adult terrain, before she entered.

After a moment of stunned silence, my mother erupted, "Amy, what are you doing? What did you tell them?"

Buoyed by the self-righteousness of a heroine who has risked all to save her brothers from a lifetime of ignorance and misery (and by the confidence that Dr. Ferdinand would take my side should my mother punish me too severely), I did the unthinkable in our family: I yelled back.

"I told them about Dad and the hospital, and I don't care what you think. Dr. Ferdinand told me. They have the right to know."

Her yell had been scary enough, but the glare that followed my outburst was chilling—reflecting, I imagined, the kind of anger and hatred that insane parents feel just before they murder their children. But that thought flickered for only a moment; after all, other than one half-hearted slap on my bottom and an intense squeeze of my arm, my mother had never touched me in anger, and neither of my parents had ever even threatened me with physical punishment. And when she barked, "Harold and Jimmy, go to your rooms right now," her glare had thawed to a look of normal parental outrage.

Not surprisingly, Harold and Jimmy hadn't needed the command; they were already scurrying to the door. She stared at me one more time and then shut the door with enough force to make clear the topic was closed—for at least the next ten years.

———

A few months later, my mother decided my therapy should end. I pleaded with her, but like a master chef reciting a recipe, she declared, "Six months is enough." *Enough for her*, I thought. In the cocoon of Dr. Ferdinand's office, for the first time safe from the risk my words might threaten a parent's stability or sobriety and relieved of the self-imposed responsibility to save my father, I had felt the first flutters of a self emerging, one that might be able to express emotions without the fear of mental illness.

But six months of therapy wouldn't be enough to counteract the contradictory message I received from my parents about how to cope with emotional problems. By age seventeen, a year after I'd stopped seeing Dr. Ferdinand, I would tell my mother I wanted to be a social worker because I enjoyed helping people. I also figured, though I didn't say it, that I'd already had valuable experience through closely observing a sober-alcoholic mother and a potentially suicidal father. And, I reassured myself, if I were the one trained to solve emotional issues, I couldn't possibly be mentally ill. It would be an immunization of sorts.

I thought she would be proud I'd arrived at this important

decision, had committed to such a compassionate and worthwhile endeavor, but instead she dismissed my plan—*"For God's sake, Amy. Why would you want to spend all day listening to people's problems?"* I dropped the idea and absorbed her implicit warning: feelings might be contagious and, in my father's case, could have dangerous consequences. A person who listened to others' problems was as weak as the person who couldn't handle them. I was deeply humiliated by her reaction, but I also thought she might be right.

My father offered very different advice. On some school nights during my later teen years, I'd find my father sitting alone at the beige-and-white-speckled Formica table in the breakfast area of our kitchen. With a yellow number one pencil in hand, he'd look up from his legal pad.

"Hey, Dad," I said one of those nights. "How's it going?" I didn't need to ask. Ever on alert, I'd noticed the struggle in his half smile.

"Well, Ame, it's hard."

I could have said, "Sorry, Dad," made an excuse, and headed for the door. But I couldn't leave him sitting there alone, looking upset. Too risky, too selfish.

"Is it your writing?" I sat to his right and glanced at the window behind him, my mother's sentry post during our childhood. From there, on late afternoons, she would call us home by blowing a whistle so commandingly that Harold, Jimmy, and I could hear it from anywhere in the neighborhood. Compared to the other mothers' signals—the clear rings of an old-fashioned teacher's handbell, the loud, om-like hums of a conch shell—our whistle jarred.

"Well, honey, it's more than that."

"Oh," was all I could manage. I wasn't sure I wanted to know what the "more" was, but I didn't get up.

"You know. When something is bothering you, you just have to dig deep. Keep at it until you get there."

I flashed on Dr. Ferdinand. *"Six months is enough, Amy,"* Mom had said.

"Like with a psychiatrist, or something?"

"Yes, Ame. Anything could be important, the answer. You have to tell them, no matter how painful." As he nodded, the overhead light flickered in his brown eyes, making them for a moment distinguishable from the dark circles underneath.

Some nights I'd ask my father a few questions, based on the unmerited confidence I'd derived from a scant six months in therapy. But mostly I'd listen. Then I'd reassure myself that I'd helped, if only by being compassionate—not like my mother, I thought, whose clenched jaws and intermittent huffs were discernible whenever she spoke to him for more than a few moments.

Perhaps my mother feared my therapy would become perpetual, as it had for my father, or raise other issues she didn't want to confront, or exacerbate my already considerable teenage moodiness, but I was certain her decision to end it was a punishment for having revealed the family secret to my brothers. I'd posed a threat to her frozen grip over the household. Years later, I would appreciate that she believed her control was vital to her sobriety and my father's mental stability. But even then, whenever I recalled her decision, my chest would sink—a sense memory of what, at the time, had felt like utter callousness.

5

OPPONENTS

MY MOTHER'S ANGRY REACTION TO MY DISCLOSURE
of the family secret had achieved its purpose—it had scared me
into silence and reestablished the status quo of family censor-
ship—but it didn't stop me from retaliating in other ways
against her. And like any adolescent at the height of her power
to infuriate a parent, I chose the perfect arena: the tennis court.

Some people look for their self-esteem, emotional well-be-
ing, and life's purpose in career or family; for my mother, that
search began again every time she opened a can of fresh tennis
balls. She had always been a talented athlete. In her junior year
of high school, her athletic prowess was interpreted as evidence
of a lack of intellectual ability, and she was moved to the "voca-
tional" (read: secretarial) track. To his credit, her father was
furious. He called up the headmistress and yelled, "If she's not
college material by now, what the hell have I been paying you for
all these years?"

My mother was quietly reassigned to the college preparatory
classes. She played golf until she was about fifteen, when her
father came home one day and announced, "Virginia, I don't
like the way those men are looking at you at the country club.
I've joined a new one, Woodstock, and you are going to play
tennis there." He handed her a tennis racket; it was the first time

she'd ever held one. If he thought he was getting her out of trouble, he was unwittingly opening her up to more.

I asked her once if she had been angry with her father for insisting she give up golf, the sport she loved most, for one she had never even played. She said, "Not at all. All I cared about was playing something."

She was naturally talented at the new game, and within a year she was the Indianapolis city novice champion. By age twenty-one, she'd won both the Indianapolis city and Indiana state championships. For a time, her doubles partner was Shirley Fry, who would later win singles titles at Wimbledon and the US, French, and Australian Opens.

By high school her two passions—tennis and alcohol—had combined nicely into a comfortable cocktail. As a solid junior player, she was frequently asked by adults to fill in as a fourth in doubles games. Afterwards, she always managed to get something from the bar poured into her Coke.

When her father thought he was paying his daughter's incidental expenses at Briarcliff Junior College, he had no idea he was paying her bar tab. The first Friday of the month, she would deposit her father's check with the local bartender to ensure that she could drink until the next one arrived. To pay for her other expenses, she wrote papers for other girls. She told me once that she sometimes charged more for C papers than A papers because they were harder to write.

Tennis would save her college career. Scheduled to graduate from junior college on a Saturday, she was told on Thursday that she, the best athlete at the school, would not walk because she had failed to satisfy the sixteen-hour physical education requirement. Not one to be deterred, she asked if she could satisfy the requirement by playing tennis for sixteen hours the next day. The dean agreed and that is what she did. She asked everyone she knew to come down to the courts the next day, and there she played a succession of opponents continuously from sunup until dark. She graduated the next day, her father—who had come from Indiana for the festivities—none the wiser.

The consequences of my mother losing a tennis match seemed, to me, to be only slightly less grave than those of upsetting my father. Within seconds of entering our house, I could tell whether she'd won or lost by the thunder of her heel pound, the snort of her smoke-filled exhale, and the intermittent "damn its." If any of us kids had been lucky enough to see each other before we saw our mother, we'd commiserate. It would be days before her mood would lighten.

I would wonder later whether her desperate need to win was not so much a reflection of her intense competitive spirit but of her determination to avoid self-pity, an opponent far more formidable than anyone who had ever stood across the net from her. My mother once told me that overcoming self-pity was the hardest part of the program for her. One of AA's many sayings, which she loved to collect and distribute—"Poor me, poor me, pour me a drink"—was a helpful reminder.

When I first heard the story about my mother's experience of losing her own mother at two years old, I imagined that was when her struggle with self-pity began.

Her first clear memory was hearing people say to her father (at the reception, since she was too young to attend the funeral), "Poor Virginia. Poor, poor Virginia." And those comments continued throughout her childhood, mothers of friends looking at her with such pity in their eyes. She had an older and a younger brother. Soon after giving birth to the baby, Tommy, their mother, Augusta Wilson Binford, contracted a breast infection and, without antibiotics, died a month later.

On her deathbed, she had a premonition. "You take care of Virginia and Tommy," she told her husband. "Frankie is coming with me." Her father would soon understand his wife's message. Frankie, his namesake, died from scarlet fever two years later.

The winter after Frankie died, my mother, struck with a dangerously high fever, almost joined him. Although her father saved her by frantically throwing her in a bath of alcohol, she would often wonder whether that cure had set the stage for another potentially fatal disease.

From then on, her father was taking no chances. The next winter, he took her and Tommy to Union Station, where he introduced them for the first time to their governess—a stern-looking middle-aged woman. He waved goodbye as the three of them boarded a train bound for the Gulf Coast town of Biloxi, Mississippi, where the mild climate, their father hoped, would protect them from illness until their return to Indianapolis in mid-spring. Poor Virginia, indeed. By her sixth birthday, she had lost her mother and brother and now had a younger brother who was too young to recognize their absence and a father whose reaction to these tragedies, though perhaps in keeping with that of other widowers of 1928, was to create more loss.

During the three or four winters my mother and her brother Tommy spent in Biloxi, it's unlikely their father could visit often, as the train trip took twenty-four hours and he had significant responsibilities in Indianapolis running two growing businesses. A few days before one of his visits (in what would turn out to be their last winter on the Gulf Coast), the governess announced that the children would be meeting their new mother. The tingles of excitement my mother usually felt at the prospect of seeing him now felt more like seismic tremors. Waiting with her brother on the steps of the Biloxi railroad station, she promised herself that she would not abandon her real mother—a vow that was immediately tested when she noticed the kindness in the face of the woman who emerged from the station on her father's arm. But she would not replace her mother yet, and when introduced to their "new mother," she extended her arm to shake hands. Expecting her brother to demonstrate the same loyalty, she shook her head in disgust as Tommy, too young to remember their "old mother," said, "Hi, Mommy," and held out his arms for a hug.

———

With my mother as our principal tennis teacher, my brothers and I inherited, to differing degrees, her competitiveness and struggle with self-pity on the court. She introduced Jimmy, Harold, and me to the game during our family's first summer in Wainscott in 1961, when we were six, seven, and eight respectively. (Louise was away at camp.) Although the small house we'd rented was outside its confines, we joined the Georgica Association, a private enclave of homeowners that bordered the 290-acre Georgica Pond on the east, the small hamlet of potato farmers on the west, and the ocean on the south. The rest of Wainscott consisted of farm fields—corn, potato, and strawberry—farmhouses, a small cemetery, a one-room schoolhouse, a post office in the front room of a crotchety old lady's house, a general store that sold milk and Coke and some penny candy, and another, much smaller, pond. The area was little known in 1961. There wasn't even a sign on the highway for Wainscott. If you didn't know where it was, you would speed right by, and that's how both the year-round and summer communities preferred it.

As my mother told it, if she was going to teach tennis to her own children, she might as well teach anyone else's who were interested too. And that's how the Georgica Association Tennis Program was started. She was a born teacher, no matter the subject. Her gift was being able to simplify the complex, whether that be the anatomy of a perfect backhand or the basics of algebra. She produced some talented players. She was also able to handle the emotional, racket-throwing ones—because, I believe, she saw herself in them. She could motivate the uncoordinated and the uncooperative. She took her role very seriously. Through tennis, she felt, she was teaching the skills essential to success and happiness in life: etiquette, honesty, teamwork, diligence, self-control, and handling defeat—the latter two of which she still struggled with herself.

Of her children, Harold was the most talented player and bore the brunt of my mother's expectations. Nevertheless, she expected me to develop a decent game and represent her well on the court. So I took lessons and played competitively on the association's team during the summer and on my high school's team in the spring.

———

One afternoon the summer after my mother ended my therapy, I was picking up a tennis ball that had rolled up against the tennis court's dark green wooden backboard when my mother suddenly appeared in the narrow entrance a few feet away from me. Whatever she said, like everything else that came out of her mouth that summer, sounded to me like the screech of a circular saw. After a quick exchange, I leaned forward and said in a voice loud enough to be heard on the next court, "I AM NEVER PLAYING TENNIS AGAIN. *EV-ER.*"

My mother would have been angry at me for raising my voice against her at home—an offense considered so grave we children rarely risked it—but to do so on a Georgica Association court where members strictly observed a Wimbledon-like silence that my mother took pains to enforce was both infuriating and humiliating. "You will regret this one day," she hissed. "You'll never be able to join a country club if you don't have a decent game."

Had she said I'd regret it because I was wasting my talent, or because I'd get fatter than I already was, perhaps I would have reconsidered for a fraction of a second. But it was 1969, and I was sixteen.

I followed her as she walked toward her car.

"Are you kidding? You think I'll ever want to be in a snobby country club like you?" And, enunciating each syllable like it was a nail to be hammered, I barked over my shoulder as I got on my bike, "I COULD NOT CARE LESS."

I hoped I'd drawn blood. Much later, I would wince at just how good it had felt to hurt her.

6

IN THE CROSSWALK AGAIN

AS NEWS OF MY TRUCK ACCIDENT SPREAD, I WOULD tell what happened over and over. My punch line—that I got hit by a truck but was more likely to die suffocating on my dry cleaning—always got a good laugh. With each retelling, I found more humor, so much so that friends apologized for laughing at my misfortune. With the episode reduced to shtick, I didn't have to think about the actual accident, or my injuries. And the fact that I'd gotten a concussion didn't seem like too big a deal. Though my doctor and Ed both urged me to see specialists, as far as I was concerned, in a week or two I would be completely back to normal, the dizziness, cloudiness, and pain notwithstanding. In the meantime, I was happy to lie in bed and chat with people who called to check in on me, a perfect excuse to do nothing at all.

Then our next-door neighbor, Pat, called. My ratio with Pat was ten to one. Ten messages on the machine to one pickup. Listening to her obsess about her favorite topics, which included caterpillar infestation, pool-cleaning tools, and the Obama stickers sprouting up in the neighborhood, was excruciating.

But that day I picked up. My appetite for sympathy and laughs apparently had no bounds. I was able to ignore what she was saying and simply focus on the way she spoke—in short bursts out of the side of her mouth, every phrase uttered with the gravity usually reserved for matters of life and death, like Jimmy Cagney before the bank heist issuing final orders to the men hunched around him. When, after an hour, it was she, not I, who was eager to hang up, I lay there stunned.

Then I called the neurologist.

———

While I knew my brain needed some attention, I was surprised when my general practitioner, who was not much of an alarmist, insisted I see an osteopath. I had no broken bones, no internal injuries, and no reason to elevate this accident to anything more than a close call accompanied by a laugh track. But, according to Dr. Cannon, even if you had no signs of broken bones, your body still required treatment after such a violent shake.

That's how I ended up going to see Dr. Friedman.

I refused Ed's offer to drive me out to the office in Montauk about thirty minutes from home, much of it within view of the ocean.

"I can drive myself out there," I said. "It's been a month."

"It's closer to three weeks," he reminded me. "You're going to have to deal with the highway. It's Friday, and weekend people are going to be speeding out there."

"Don't be ridiculous. It's no big deal." I wanted to be back to normal, and if that meant pretending that driving was easy for me, that's what I would do.

A week after the accident, the police had asked me to come down to the station to be interviewed. It could wait a few weeks, they said, if I wasn't up to it yet. Although I wasn't too steady on

my feet, I wanted to go immediately. A sure sign of getting back
to normal. I let Matt do me the favor of driving, but even as a
passenger I was scared. I adjusted the radio and looked no higher
than the dashboard. I couldn't shake the feeling that other cars
on the road might suddenly swerve into us.

As I drove out to Montauk, I thought Ed might have been
right. Several times, I pulled over to the gravelly shoulder and
watched the oncoming traffic. I nodded as each passing car
stayed obediently in its lane and hoped I could reeducate myself
for reentry into the world, where I once again could take my
safety for granted.

Dr. Friedman was the first complete stranger to whom I told
the story of the accident. I gave him the shtick and got a few
chuckles, but he already knew what I did not: even the most
well-honed stand-up routine can't keep a victim of such an accident from eventually facing the fact that she's experienced a
trauma.

As Dr. Friedman gently pressed a few places at the base of
my skull, electricity buzzed through my body, just as it had as I
lay in the street. Suddenly, I was back in the crosswalk. With no
warning, and for the first time since the accident, I began to cry.
Although I despised breaking down in front of strangers, I could
have stopped the tears about as well as I could have stopped the
truck.

"Oh God, Dr. Friedman, there was nothing I could do. It just
kept coming. I was hurt. Really hurt." I swallowed a sob as tears
curled around my ears and dripped onto the fresh white sheet
underneath me.

Until that moment, I'd been able to do what I'd always done
—avoid feelings of vulnerability by minimizing them or resort-

ing to humor. For me, fending off helplessness had become almost reflexive. Though I couldn't say what frightened me so much, the danger of giving in to that helplessness felt undeniably real, just like the trapdoors of my childhood. But lying in that office, I was suddenly defenseless, overwhelmed by how completely frightened and alone I had felt on that street.

"Yes, Amy, you were hurt," he said. "Please don't downplay your experience."

I might as well have been lying there naked. I grabbed for cover. "I mean, not badly hurt, Dr. Friedman. I mean, I'm so lucky. I could have been killed. It's just a concussion. Some dizziness."

I was relieved when he changed the subject. He said he hadn't noticed any significant changes in my nervous system as I'd recounted the story and "reexperienced" the accident. He speculated, based on my relative calm, that I had likely avoided more serious injury because I hadn't tensed at the time of impact.

"I did just kind of surrender," I confessed. "I gave up. Right before it hit me."

"Interesting. That must have helped. Any idea why you were able to do that?"

How could I, as a mother, admit that I had been willing, if only for a moment, to let go of my sons—that I'd been relieved to be free of the fear that no matter how hard I tried not to, I would pass on the emotional legacy of my childhood?

Instead, I came up with a more plausible, or at least less maternally damning, explanation and suggested that as I'd been doing Transcendental Meditation for the last thirty-five years, perhaps my nervous system was accustomed to settling down, even under stress.

7

MEDITATION

DURING HIGH SCHOOL, I COULDN'T HAVE PREDICTED
that my brother Harold would be the one to introduce our family
to Transcendental Meditation. By then, his drinking and drug
use already had a desperate, determined quality, different from
the usual teenage experimentation. He would try anything and
was brazen in doing so—sometimes in his room at the top of the
back stairs, out of earshot of my parents' bedroom. While pot
was just becoming popular in our high school at that time and
some kids were moving into psychedelics, Harold was one of the
very few who snorted heroin. How he did this and maintained
good enough grades to get into Harvard was hard to fathom.

My mother may have been too preoccupied at that time
with other potential dangers that faced Harold to notice his sub-
stance abuse. For example, she forbade him from applying to
Yale—where, if accepted, he would be the fourth generation of
Turners to attend. She was concerned that my father (Class of
'37) would, whether consciously or unconsciously, impose the
same unrealistic expectations and pressures onto his son that his
father had placed on him and his brother—gaining admission
into Yale's most exclusive social club and earning a varsity "Y," to
name just two—a subject so painful that my father was still writing about it forty years later.

My mother had long ago admitted her own problem with alcohol, but she still suffered from the disease of denial at this stage in Harold's drinking. She would later laugh when she told me the story of the day she noticed the police trailing her as she drove the car that Harold and I usually drove. When she pulled over to find out what the problem was, the policeman apologized, "Sorry, Mrs. Turner, we thought it was Harold."

She laughed; I cringed. It was obvious to me they suspected drug possession or open containers of alcohol and were looking for an excuse to pull him over.

Although Harold still lived at home, my mother seemed oblivious to what I knew from a thousand miles away in Switzerland, where I was spending the year between high school and college (1971–72). Thanks to letters from Mrs. Ribner, our eleventh-grade English teacher, it was clear that Harold was heading for disaster.

According to one letter, there were "a lot of rumors floating about Harold's being a drug addict—not just pot or hash but harder stuff—speed, LSD, etc. . . . It's known that Harold hangs around with what is considered unsavory company: [with] the biggest drug pusher, etc. . . . Kids were saying he's *shooting* speed. . . . [The basketball coach] said he was worried about Harold's peculiar behavior, tired, absent, late, game not as good, etc. . . ." There was nothing I could do from Switzerland except worry and write angry letters to Harold with the ineffective pleas of an adolescent to "stop being stupid, don't get into trouble, Mom's going to kill you."

Much later, I would question a teacher's judgment in sharing such distressing news with a teenager who—in the pre-Internet days, when mail could take weeks and transatlantic phone calls were expensive—was so far removed from the support of close friends and family. But in fact, Mrs. Ribner wasn't much older than her students.

That should have been obvious to me the first time I saw her walking down the aisle in the high school auditorium in 1968— almost six feet tall, long brown hair, wearing partially shaded aviator glasses, a dark tan suede miniskirt, a tight narrow-ribbed black turtleneck, and high-heeled, over-the-knee boots.

Mrs. Ribner's glamour, intelligence, and youth made her incredibly alluring to most of her students, but she admitted only a few into her entourage. Harold and I were both flattered to be included in the group, which meant we enjoyed her undivided attention in school and could call her by her first name, Patsy, off school grounds. At her wedding—a glittering affair in a ballroom at The Plaza Hotel that I attended while still in high school—I sat, mesmerized, along with about two hundred other guests. Several times, she invited a few of her students to join her for dinner. Sitting around a fondue pot on the floor of her Greenwich Village apartment felt like the epitome of cool.

Yet there may have been more to our connection to Mrs. Ribner than just teenage infatuation. Perhaps Harold and I felt she recognized something special in each of us that our parents' attention, which was little more than monitoring, did not usually convey, or we recognized in her that same deeply rooted dedication to literature and writing we'd known since childhood, as familiar to us as the sound of our father's voice. Though Mrs. Ribner, as demanding of herself and her students as any English teacher could be, approached the topic with none of the angst that it caused our father.

Unfortunately, neither I nor Mrs. Ribner, nor anyone else

for that matter, had any influence over Harold's conduct. If he could graduate high school and continue with this behavior at Harvard without any ramifications, did I really need to worry about him?

Whether or not he was ready to admit he had a drinking or drug problem, I do know that emotional issues were on his mind. On one trip home together from college, in 1973 probably, he smiled at me as he pounded the steering wheel and mimicked the slight British accent of the singer on the radio, *"But then they sent me away to teach me how to be"*—he used the heel of his hand to emphasize the final words—*"sensible, logical, responsible, practical . . . dependable, clinical, intellectual, cynical . . ."* Unselfconscious about being slightly tone deaf, Harold sang on louder, but plaintively, *"At night, when all the world's asleep, the questions run too deep for such a simple man. Won't you please, please tell me what we've learned. I know it sounds absurd. But please tell me who I am."*

He turned to me then, shaking his head slightly, his smile collapsing into a sigh. "I love that song, Ame. You should get it. It's 'The Logical Song.'"

———

Later that year, as Harold told it, he noticed a group of students in his philosophy class who—unlike everyone else at Harvard, or at least unlike his circle of friends—always looked rested, clear-eyed, and happy. When he asked them why, they said they'd started Transcendental Meditation. Wanting that clarity and peace (and, though he didn't say it at that time, sobriety), he started right away. Eventually, he pestered our parents so relentlessly to learn TM that they started it too, by going to the White Plains TM Center for four consecutive evenings to learn how to meditate.

My mother was skeptical about TM, to say the least, but her doubts vanished the first time she played tennis after meditating: her depth perception and reflexes had improved so much she could practically see the gleam of another silver trophy. From then on, she meditated for twenty minutes twice a day until the day she died of lung cancer in Sloan Kettering twenty-five years later. (Although TM was a great help to her tennis game, it had done nothing for her smoking habit.)

Within weeks of learning to meditate, my mother convinced Louise, Jim, and me to learn too. I don't know how she influenced them, but for me her tactic was to drive up to Cape Cod, where I was living that summer, lend me a car for the upcoming school year, and give me a check for $150 to cover the TM initiation fees for both me and my boyfriend. Very persuasive.

I was initiated in an upstairs room that overlooked a lake surrounded by woods, no houses in sight—a view that was, by itself, meditative. As I sat for the first time, I descended into a place inside me of complete safety and peace. It was familiar as a matter of instinct, not personal experience. When later I heard that feeling described as one of "Mother being at home," I agreed that perfectly described what I'd felt.

And I did see, for a while at least, a big difference in Harold. With my parents' blessing and financial support, he took time off during his sophomore year of college in 1974 to become a TM teacher. When he returned from teacher training in Switzerland, he had cut his hair and was dressed in the informal uniform of that position: a dark gray or black suit, tie, and white shirt. Having, I believe, totally given up using alcohol and drugs, his social life mainly involved leading residence courses or watching tapes of Maharishi with other meditators.

Attending Harold's TM lectures, where his intelligence, humor, charm, and good looks were in abundant display, I was both happy for him and terribly jealous. By the time we reached our mid-twenties, however, Harold had begun drinking again and I'd decided that if having his prodigious gifts meant also having his addiction, I would opt for my mediocre endowment.

Even when he was drinking, Harold continued to insist that practicing TM and following an Ayurvedic health regimen would take care of his problem. AA, the obvious alternative, probably posed too many emotional conflicts. For a young man who was trying to establish an independent identity, it might have been too threatening to seek help from an organization in which his mother played an active role. By that time our mother was twenty-five years sober and highly respected in the program for the number of people she had helped and her straightfor-ward yet perceptive explanations of the principles. Even if Harold had avoided meetings in the areas where "Virginia T." was well known, which included suburban New York, the Hamptons, and Key West, where she spent a few months each winter, I imagine it would have been difficult for him not to feel her presence—or judgment. But when the question of attending meetings came up, he didn't share those feelings, if he'd had them. Instead, he was likely to taunt her, "You were drinking at my age. I'll stop drinking when you did, when I'm thirty-five. Leave me alone."

8

———

LAUGH LINES

DETERMINED NOT TO LET MY VERTIGO AND PERSISTENT
headache interfere with my usual activities, I spent most of the
summer after the accident trying to reassure myself and others
that I was "back to normal." Ed asked me whether it might be too
much for me to teach and take on the teachers' union copresi-
dency, a position I'd assumed toward the close of the previous
school year. Absolutely not, I told him. I had made a commitment, and I would keep my word. But perhaps my insistence had
less to do with integrity than clinging to an illusion of indispens-
ability or a facade of personal strength.

Thus I found myself lying in bed and arguing over the
phone with the superintendent about sick leave policy or class
sizes or whatever topic arose that summer. Fortunately, my co-
president handled much of the work, but I never refused a task.
"No, Nancy, really. I feel fine; I'll go to the meeting."

In late July of 2010, just two weeks after the accident, I sat
with the union labor relations specialist and two custodians at
student desks arranged in a small circle in a corner of the seventh-grade English classroom. (The teachers' union was responsible for negotiating the custodians' contract.) Crisply dressed in
a navy skirt and white short-sleeved shirt, a light beige cotton
cardigan draped over my shoulders (just in case the air-condi-

tioning worked), I tried to look the part. I nodded periodically and tried to use high vocabulary to disguise how slowly I was processing the conversation.

Any time I glanced down at my notes, or at the men to my left or right, I felt like I was spinning. The only way I knew to stop that sensation was to grab my head with both hands, a non-verbal signal to my vestibular system that I was stationary, but that gesture would hardly be professional—so, as inconspicuously as possible, I propped my elbow on the desk, rested my chin in my cupped palm, and pressed my fingers into my cheek until my brain got the message.

At the end of the meeting, our labor representative remarked that she was surprised I had been well enough to attend a meeting so soon after my accident. Her quizzical expression made me pause. I was surprised for a different reason. The option of staying home and resting had never occurred to me. I was not sick, I said to myself.

———

In early August I volunteered to be the teacher representative at a meeting of the Committee on Special Education. I happened to enter the building just as the seventh grader whose educational placement was the subject of the meeting arrived with his mother. We made small talk as we walked together down the hall. They were nervous about the meeting; I, feeling dizzy, was nervous about losing my balance and bumping into them. I used the square linoleum floor tiles as a guide, making sure to step only in the same two contiguous rows so that I would walk in a straight line.

As soon as I entered the room, I knew this meeting would be far more difficult than I had anticipated. Unlike our usual special education meetings, where at most five people (and rarely any psychiatrists) attended, seven others were sitting at student desks arranged in a conference-table shape. The student's psychiatrist sat at one end, the school's principal at the other. Seated on either side were the director of special education, guidance counselor, school psychologist, and two other teachers.

The tension was palpable. The parents were seeking an unusual and expensive accommodation for their son that the school principal, with precedent and budget on his mind, was reluctant to grant. The other school personnel, including me, would be caught in the middle. I had rehearsed what I intended to say, but now I wondered whether it would sound professional enough, especially to a psychiatrist who might question me. As I mulled over how to improve my comments, I lost track of the discussion. I was unable to hold two thoughts at once, a multitasking skill that before the accident would have come easily to me.

I gave my rehearsed comments and was relieved when I wasn't asked any follow-up questions. When other observations occurred to me, I would miss the opportunity to share them. I felt like a New York City tourist who carefully positions herself so that she can elbow her way into the arriving subway but then somehow, inexplicably, gets distracted and looks up moments later to see the train screech away.

I spent most of the meeting trying to look professionally engaged and listening as the conversations sped by.

———

In addition to suggesting I see an osteopath for physical manipulation, my general practitioner had recommended I see a therapist to forestall the possibility of developing severe or prolonged symptoms of PTSD.

Since the accident, I had stopped jaywalking, and I never started into a crosswalk unless the car was fully stopped and I could see the driver return my wave. On a trip to do errands in the village one day, Ed dashed across the street, expecting me to follow as usual. When, after waiting for the light to change, I finally reached him, he was shocked to see tears dripping down my cheeks. I was embarrassed, but like an abandoned toddler, I couldn't contain my reaction: "Jesus, Ed, are you trying to kill me? I can't do that anymore."

As far as I was concerned, crossing the street with added caution was perfectly understandable. I wasn't experiencing sudden flashbacks or feelings of panic, and I was aware of the research on TM's beneficial effects on veterans suffering from PTSD, so I wasn't worried about developing the full-blown disorder. But just to make sure, I did think it might be a good idea to talk to someone. I could hear my father's voice: "Whatever it is, Ame, you just have to dig deep."

I made an appointment with Barbara, a therapist I'd seen a few years before on a regular basis. We met weekly throughout the summer and then occasionally thereafter. I recounted the accident during many of those visits, but as she would point out to me later, I could never do so without including jokes. She didn't suggest that I drop the humor, probably aware that I wasn't ready to confront feelings of helplessness and fear.

———

Toward the end of the summer, Dr. Friedman recommended that I take a leave of absence from school and return in the new year. But I wouldn't consider it. I worried that if I was home for that long, I would have to acknowledge to others, and more importantly to myself, that I had been injured and was too vulnerable and weak to soldier on.

Dr. Friedman suggested that perhaps I could handle starting school in September if I got permission to teach fewer classes and to lie down and rest in a dark, quiet room in between them. It was obvious to me that Dr. Friedman had no experience with an underfunded, overcrowded public school. As a compromise, I took a six-week leave and planned to return in mid-October to teach the required number of classes, between which I would sit in a noisy, moldy basement faculty room, all the while willing away the dizziness and pain. I was not sick, I reassured myself.

9

BLACKOUT

I WAS ONE OF THOSE OBNOXIOUS COLLEGE STUDENTS who worried that she'd flunked a test or bombed a paper only to blush when she received an A.

My worst experience came during my freshman year in 1972, in Religion 101, with the first paper I was assigned. Each time I sat down to type, after obsessively positioning the paper in the roller until it was perfectly straight across, then twisting the roller back and forth until three inches of white paper appeared, checking the ribbon a few times, and placing my now inky fingers expectantly on the keyboard, I pressed no keys. Despite having conducted hours of research, I was convinced that whatever I wrote about the New Testament would be laughably wrong. I stared at the blank page, paralyzed between the only two choices I could envision: write a paper that would expose me as an idiot or blow it off and admit I was emotionally incapable of coping with even the routine academic pressure of college.

In the beginning I would just get up and take a walk— maybe down the hall to flop on a friend's bed and spill out my woes. As the deadline approached, I'd force myself to sit at the typewriter and then start breathing so fast I couldn't think. Now it was too embarrassing to confide in anyone. I couldn't sleep, and taking nips of my roommate's Galliano, a syrupy yellow liqueur, no longer worked. (Despite my roommate's great annoyance, I consumed the entire bottle.) I couldn't do anything except sit in classes and pretend I was listening. Surely I was going to flunk out, going to be exposed as unqualified—if not for lack of intelligence, then, like my father, for being too emotionally unstable.

I told my professors I wasn't feeling well, alluded to a "nervous breakdown" without using the term, and drove home. Thank God my father was away that week. For sure he would have recognized the signs and scared me into having the real thing.

Although I was surprised that my mother was so calm about all this, perhaps I shouldn't have been. After all, she wouldn't have asked me what was wrong. She always avoided the discussion of difficult feelings, an approach I usually found cold and insensitive. But on this occasion, it was the perfect maternal response. Years later I would recall this incident when I came across what appeared to be a draft for one of her talks on AA, in which she wrote, "'Pain,' like 'depression,' is a dead-end word. Our program is an action program."

That weekend, she suggested I sit at the largest desk in the house (ironically, my father's desk, already so accustomed to anxious writers) and just try. Which I did. She even brought me bowls of mint chocolate chip ice cream—unheard of for a mother who monitored her daughters' weights as obsessively as her own. I think we pretended I just had a bad cold.

Finally, I wrote the paper. My professor gave it an A but commented in the margin, "Amy, please don't use erasable paper again."

———

In my sophomore year, my mother's prescription for action was far less helpful to me. I was struggling with whether to transfer to a different college. The decision should have been fairly straightforward: just weigh the pros and cons. But the only pro on the list was being able to live with my new bass player boyfriend in Boston.

I knew I was about to make an important choice based on neediness. My boyfriend, whose temper was starting to trouble me, was exerting more pressure, signaling that he'd break up with me if I didn't transfer. I was panicked, as if without the gravitational pull of the relationship I'd somehow hurtle off into space, and my reaction was almost as upsetting to me as the potential breakup.

The deadline for transfer applications was looming. I should have known better than to call my mother, but I was desperate for advice. If I did what an adult told me to do, I hoped maybe I'd feel like one myself.

The black rotary phone was attached to the wall in my bedroom. Mom answered and accepted the charges for the collect call. I was glad of the phone's coiled cord that, fully outstretched, allowed me to pace a large swath of the room.

After we exchanged hellos and I explained why I was calling on a Wednesday, rather than the usual Sunday, my mother hesitated.

"So, what's the problem, Amy, just transfer."

"Yeah, Mom, but academically it's probably a bad decision. At this late stage, I probably won't be able to get into as good a school."

No answer. Just the static created by her breathing.

"And Bob is really pressuring me . . . I don't know him that well . . ." I don't know if she heard my voice crack. I faked a cough.

"Amy, *just make a decision.*"

"Oh." My face flushed. I shouldn't have been surprised that she cut me off rather than listen to a catalog of confused feelings. "Okay, so it doesn't matter to you?"

I can't be sure whether she began her response with, "For God's sake," but I hear those words now, her code for STOP TALKING. I do know she said, "Stay in Connecticut or move to Boston. I've got to go."

I hung up and burst into tears. Maybe I hadn't made it clear how upset I was, but I think she knew. She may have decided it best to treat me like an adult capable of making her own decisions. Or, given my father's seemingly ever-present emotional issues, she may have simply lacked the capacity to deal with mine. In any case, she couldn't help me, and I did what any insecure adolescent with questionable self-esteem would do: I moved to Boston.

———

Regular classes at Boston University were generally less rigorous for me than my classes at Connecticut College had been, so I had a reprieve from academic worry until the first semester of my senior year—when, based on a professor's recommendation and my grade point average, I was invited to do distinction work, a prerequisite for graduating summa cum laude. I was terrified of the possibility of failing, and the only professor available to be my mentor was curt and cold, unlikely to offer any support through what would undoubtedly be an anxiety-laden process. I got as far as buying the textbook for the statistics class he said I was required to take. I opened it, immediately saw the F I would surely get, and burst into tears.

Later, the professor just stared at me, his eyebrows raised, as I sniffled and swallowed back tears and told him I just couldn't handle the pressure.

I would graduate magna cum laude instead, and my mother, whose pride was undeniable and reassuring, would be the only member of the family to attend my graduation.

———

If college had been anxiety provoking, my first two years of law school were like going through a meat grinder. I felt sure they would squeeze the pretense out of me, exposing me for the inferior intellect I was.

Home for Thanksgiving break in 1976 during my first year of law school in New York City, I was already panicking about flunking out. It wasn't totally a product of my homegrown worry; we had been told on the first day to look left and then right, because one of the three of us wouldn't return second semester. And it certainly didn't help when my father asked me how it was going.

"Um, pretty well, Dad. It's tough, though." I was practiced by then in how to discuss worrisome topics with my father. Confiding some unhappiness or psychological struggle was the best way to connect with him. He could relate to that. After all, anxiety and depression were his expertise, his life's work. But I had to be careful. Too much and he would grab and internalize it, and who knew what he might do next. As my mother always warned, "He's sick, don't get him upset, he can't handle it."

So, after sharing a small dose of my worry, I reassured him, "But it's okay. It's hard, but I can handle it."

"I don't know how you do it, Ame," he said.

So far, so good. I hadn't crossed the line my mother had so clearly drawn for us. But I wasn't prepared for what came next.

"You know, I really *don't* know how you do it," he continued. "I don't know if you knew this, but I tried it once, Ame. Just couldn't do it. First year. It was bad, honey. I left."

I didn't know, and it stopped me cold. Today, I don't recall whether he actually used the phrase "flunked out." It didn't matter. Either alternative—incapable of doing the work or of just handling the pressure—was equally threatening. Like father, like daughter. There was no escaping it, no stopping it, like a boulder already halfway to the bottom.

———

I did survive that first year of law school, but it took a lot of white-knuckling, jaw clenching, and the distraction of falling in love with Ed to get me through.

The relationship with my musician boyfriend started unraveling during my senior year in college after I refused to apply to law schools in Boston, and it was basically over by the time I started law school. I noticed Ed on the first day of orientation and was instantly attracted to him. (I also noticed the woman sitting beside him and duly noted that she was far thinner and cooler than me, but fantasized that they were just then ending their relationship.)

Ed was tall, dark, and handsome, but not in the way that phrase conjures. His mustache drooped around the edges of his mouth, his hair fell a couple of inches over his collar, and his brown leather bomber jacket and jeans didn't scream "lawyer." And although someone might have thought he resembled the proverbial bad boy, they wouldn't have been looking closely enough. I knew instantly that he was kind—"instinctively kind," as my father would say in his wedding toast to us five years later. There was something about his brown eyes: a softness, a warmth that could never give way to the barracuda stare I associated with lawyers and businessmen. Eventually, I would see the same expression in his mother, who would prove to me that unconditional love was not a myth.

Ed and I spoke to each other for the first time two days after I first saw him, when I turned around to find him behind me in a line of students waiting to buy law books. I'm sure I couldn't hide the blush of excitement, and he looked somewhat nervous as well.

"Hey, first year?" I asked as nonchalantly as I could.

"Yup. Getting books, if there are any left by the time we get there."

"Where're you from?"

"Outside New York."

"Oh, where?"

"Uh, just north of the city."

"Far?"

"Not really."

It was obvious he didn't want to tell me, but now I was curious. I recognized the tactics I would use to avoid admitting that I'd grown up in Bronxville, a wealthy, white enclave well known in the metropolitan area for its snobbery and prejudice. "Yeah, me too. Westchester County?"

"Uh, yeah." He was now looking at his feet.

"Hey, look. I'm from Bronxville. There is nowhere more embarrassing than that. Come on. Where are you from?"

He laughed. "Okay, I'll tell you: Irvington."

More bucolic than Bronxville, and set on the Hudson River, Irvington was more economically if not racially diverse than Bronxville.

We'd grown up twenty minutes away from each other; our high schools were even in the same football league.

Over the next six weeks, I thought I'd also be able to nudge Ed into asking me out. Lucky for me, Ed's last name started with an *R* and mine with a *T,* which meant we were in Section C, the students who were at the end of the alphabet and had identical class schedules. But after many lingering conversations before and after class, supposedly chance meetings in the library, and suspiciously synchronized cravings for a bagel from Gil's, the small coffee place next to the bookstore, I hadn't been successful.

Thank God for the alphabetized seating charts of law school; Ed's assigned seat was right behind mine. One Friday afternoon, just as torts class was beginning, I turned around to ask him, as casually as I could, "Hey, feel like getting a drink after class?"

"Sure."

That drink lasted well into the night, and marked the beginning of what would become a lifelong relationship.

———

One evening during the summer after our first year, we sat on a bench in Washington Square Park.

"I'm going to be better second year," I told Ed. "I don't think I'm going to be such a wreck. I think I'll get a handle on it."

"I hope so. You really worried a lot this year."

"I know, I know. Jesus. Remember when I couldn't sleep and kept missing Civil Procedure? I thought I was going to fail it."

"Yeah, but of course you got a B. You did well."

"I know, but this panic just comes over me. I feel like if I make a mistake or something, I'm going to die."

"What? Really? Have you ever talked to anyone about it?"

"Like who?" I was getting a little suspicious now.

"Like maybe a therapist or somebody."

I reminded him that I'd seen a therapist when I was fifteen, a story I'd told him when we were first getting to know each other.

"Yeah, I remember. But it might help for you to see someone now. Talk about what's bothering you in law school."

By now I was breathing so hard I thought I'd start snorting, too fast to keep smoking the cigarette I was holding. I stomped it out. "Ed, I am *not sick*. I do not need to see a shrink."

"I didn't say you *were* sick. A lot of people see therapists. I'm seeing one. It just helps you figure things out—bad patterns, things like that."

I got up quickly—almost a jump, because my feet thudded on the sidewalk. The sound reminded me of my mother pounding down the hall, cigarette smoke trailing behind her, saying, "Dad's sick, Amy, don't bother him with that. He'll get too upset."

"I AM NOT SICK."

"Okay, Amy, okay. Forget it. Nobody is calling you sick."

"Good, because I'm not mentally ill. I'm okay."

We were quiet then. Enough said. I shook out a Marlboro. I didn't bother to tap the pack. Seemed pretentious and took way too long when you smoked incessantly. It was usually an archaeological dig to find matches in the layers of crap in my purse, but in that moment I didn't fumble around; I seemed to know where they were, just as I knew that I was not sick, was not my father's daughter.

Suddenly, I felt a shadow at my back. Ed must have felt it too because we looked over our shoulders at the same time—and saw that the city to the north of us had gone completely dark. Before we could say anything, we turned just in time to see the lights go out in the south as well, as though southern Manhattan had been connected to one switch and someone had pulled it.

We quickly decided to go to a friend's apartment. It was a walk that would ordinarily have taken us five minutes and was one we knew well, but after fifteen minutes of stumbling around in the dark (in those pre–cell phone days, without "flashlights" in hand), we gave up and, unnerved, just headed north.

Like many New Yorkers, I was already on edge with the serial killer Son of Sam on the loose, violent crime on the increase, and the city facing a severe economic crisis. That made the eighty-block walk home in a pitch-black New York City—no lights anywhere, not in buildings, streetlamps, or traffic signals—all the more terrifying. There were no police in sight, and although I was grateful to be with Ed, I doubted he could defend us against a mugging or more dangerous attack.

The anxiety was palpable, and it would only get worse. By morning, the fact that it was ninety degrees and there was no air-conditioning anywhere was the least of it. We woke up to reports of rampant looting and news that a shooting had occurred in the pharmacy across the street in my otherwise safe Upper West Side neighborhood.

After lots of calling around, Ed and I were lucky enough to get a ride out of New York.

Under ordinary circumstances, I might have dismissed Ed's opinion that I needed therapy—but having been punctuated by a twenty-five-hour power outage that crippled the entire city of New York, our conversation was impossible for me to ignore. And although this was incredibly egocentric, I saw the blackout as a sign: *If you thought staying in the dark was comfortable, well, here's the real thing.*

When the lights came back on, I called a therapist.

———

By the following summer I had gained some self-awareness, but not enough to stanch the flood of anxiety I felt almost every day as a summer associate at a prominent Wall Street law firm.

The worst episode revolved around a speech I was asked to write for a senior partner. I was too embarrassed to admit that I knew nothing about the topic, current issues in municipal bonds, and was highly unlikely to be able to write something worthy of an experienced legal mind. I was walking down the hall when another partner casually asked me how the speech was going. I heard his first few words, but then, although his mouth continued to move, the sounds seemed to dissolve before they reached me. His forehead crinkled as he waited for my response. I opened my mouth, but I couldn't think, couldn't even retrieve the simplest response like "okay" or "fine," couldn't even look away from his expression of growing concern.

He moved a little closer—"Amy?"—but I just stood there and stared.

As he walked away, I began to defrost, feeling for the first time my racing pulse and the beads of sweat at my hairline. *Oh God*, I thought. *Is that what it's like to be catatonic?*

———

On one weekend visit to my family's house in Wainscott during the summer after law school graduation, Ed and I came home from a late Saturday night dinner. I turned the front doorknob slowly to avoid waking my mother, but before the door was even half-open, I could hear her shouting. She was already planted on the landing that overlooked the small vestibule.

"Amy, what did you do? What did you say to him?"

I could barely register all of it at once—her flaming cheeks, shooting glare, rising chest.

"How could you? I've told you so many times . . ."

I remembered Ed was with me, which was both embolden-ing and embarrassing.

"What are you talking abou—"

"Dad, Dad . . . He's so upset, it's . . ." The rest of her sentence was garbled in her sputter.

My father was in Bangladesh doing research for a book he was writing, an interest that had resulted from a job he'd had overseeing the distribution of books to a public library in Dacca.

I tried again. "I don't know what you are—"

"The letter. You told him about Harold's drinking. He might come home now. I don't even know what he's going to do now, he's so worried."

I looked over my shoulder at Ed, whose eyes widened in response. I raised my palms. Turning back to my mother, I shot each word at her. "You are out of your mind. I didn't write any letter, and I don't know who did." I brushed past Ed, and he followed me as I crunched across the driveway gravel to the car. We drove to the beach and talked—long enough for me to calm down and for my mother, we hoped, to fall asleep.

———

When she heard me getting coffee the next morning, my mother appeared in the kitchen doorway. After audibly exhaling, she said, without warmth, "I'm sorry I blamed you. I know now it wasn't you."

She wasn't sorry about yelling, just about yelling at the wrong person.

"Well," I said stiffly, "you should have found that out before screaming at me."

I wanted to add, but didn't, "Don't you think I've already learned not to take the risk of upsetting him?" It had been more than twenty years since my father had stepped onto that ledge, and yet we still behaved as though that threat were imminent. Like lab rats, we had been conditioned to respond to a trigger in the same way each time. In our family's case, we would all worry about my father's mental state, and our mother would use her anger to protect us all.

———

After graduating from a less-than-top-tier law school in 1979, I was fortunate to be offered an associate's position by a large and prestigious New York City law firm. When I told people where I'd be working, their admiration was flattering, but it did little to bolster my confidence. The work was difficult enough, but fighting my anxiety was even more exhausting—like playing an endless game of Whac-A-Mole.

In the world of large firms, new associates were expected to stay a minimum of two years, which meant for me sticking it out until September of 1981. My second year at the firm passed quickly, as Ed and I were preoccupied with planning our wedding, which would take place on a late afternoon on a sunny Saturday in July.

On our two-week honeymoon in Europe, we experienced a freedom neither of us had felt since the year we spent there in college—I in Switzerland and Ed in France. From the beginning of our relationship, we'd fantasized about leading a more unconventional life, free of the strictures of the legal and business world. In the past, those conversations had always trailed off into wistful sighs and never resulted in any action, but now, with our futures bound together, we were secure enough to take such a leap. We decided to quit our jobs in the fall (at my two-year anniversary with the firm) and live in the house my mother owned in Wainscott until we figured out how to actualize our dream life.

I was absolutely anxiety-free during those months we spent in Wainscott; I almost didn't recognize myself. We lived in a fantasy—no obligations, no worries. But frugal as we were, by the spring we needed money, and having failed to conceive of an alternative that afforded us both freedom and sufficient income, we resigned ourselves to resuming the practice of law.

Our new jobs enabled us to purchase a tiny fixer-upper in a different area of East Hampton; eventually, we'd move back to Wainscott and into a modest house we'd build next door to my mother—by which point there would rarely be any talk between us of leading an unconventional life.

I joined a five-attorney general practice in Riverhead, hoping it would be less stressful for me, but even at a small firm I was as anxious as ever. Surrounded by towers of open law books (a monument to my insecurity if ever there was one), I'd become desperate to find the answer I was looking for, scanning the pages, hoping the next sentence would read, "Amy, here it is. This is it—you've found it! *Stop worrying!*"

I didn't stop searching until the words slid around the page so fast my eyes could no longer focus. And then I'd get up to talk to Ed.

Lucky for me, Ed's first-floor law office at Legal Services overlooked my firm's parking lot. His window was just within reach if I stood on my toes. So, rather than risk the embarrassment of asking the receptionist to put me through to Ed yet again, I would often run outside and tap on the glass.

He would swivel around in his chair and open the window.

"How many days do I have to respond to a petition?"

"Amy, I told you, twenty days unless service was by nail and mail."

"I know, but do you think that rule applies to that client I told you about?"

"Yes, why wouldn't it?"

"But there could be an exception in my case. I haven't read everything—only those two treatises and the cases going back twenty years or so."

"There's no exception, I promise you. The landlord-tenant law is very clear—it's right there in RPAPL 735."

"I know, but if I'm wrong, I could screw up the whole case." By then, I'd be short of breath, like I'd just finished a 10K.

"Ame, you've got to relax. I'm telling you. Stop worrying about it and just do it."

"Okay, okay, I know." But by the time I'd walked the short distance back to my office, I was worried.

———

One night after a similar exchange, this time at the dining room table, Ed shook his head slowly, a hint of a smile about his eyes, and asked, "Have you ever heard of the word 'perseveration'?"

"No." It didn't sound very flattering, but Ed was never mean.

"It's when people keep repeating the same thing over and over. They can't stop. You know that place for the developmentally disabled where I worked before law school? There was a guy who kept frantically repeating that he'd lost his wallet. The only way to stop him was to take him outside and put him on the swing. Another guy would keep grunting and then—"

"Okay," I interrupted. "I get it. You don't have to tell me about any more mental patients."

We were laughing, but we both knew there was no swing in the world that was going to calm me down.

———

The obvious solution would have been to leave the practice of law, to acknowledge that I didn't like being a lawyer, to admit that the pressure was too intense. But to leave law would have meant to fail, to finally admit I was unable to handle what I considered the real world. Just like my father after all. And so I spent many of those years perseverating, calling Ed, and telling my therapist that I wanted to be free of anxiety, happy in a law firm—just like on *L.A. Law*, I would laugh, often through tears.

10

ONE STEP AWAY

WHEN ED AND I RETURNED TO WAINSCOTT IN 1986,
it was as my mother's next-door neighbors. By this point, my
parents—after years of barely spending any time together—had
formally divorced. My mother had given us the vacant lot ad-
joining her property to build a house on. By August of that year,
Ed and I found ourselves in a race between the completion of
our new home and the arrival of our first child. We rushed the
builder and were lucky to be able to move in a few weeks before
the birth.

But I suppose we rushed Matthew as well. Concerned that
he was two weeks late and that I'd gained more than fifty
pounds, my doctor strongly advised against waiting any longer
for labor to begin naturally. Nervous, I consented to an induced
labor, and after fourteen hours Matt was born via a C-section,
weighing in at ten pounds, two ounces. When the doctor called
out, "We have a power forward," I beamed and the attendants
cheered.

Yet within minutes, I was distraught. As the nurse whisked
Matthew away from me, the doctor announced that because I
had a fever, Matt and I had to be separated immediately. Being
cut off from him was too much to bear. When I started yelling
through sobs that I had to see my baby, they agreed to wheel my

gurney through the nursery to the NICU, where I glimpsed Matt for a few precious seconds, his chubby body squeezed into an incubator designed for preemies. I had given birth but felt like I'd already failed the most fundamental responsibility of a mother: to protect her child.

———

They separated me from Matthew due to my fever, but it turned out I'd begun losing blood (due to previously undiagnosed anemia) shortly after my delivery. With the AIDS epidemic raging, doctors were reluctant to order a transfusion for fear of giving me tainted blood. As I lay in a pain-medication-and-exhaustion-induced stupor, I felt nurses periodically nudging and pushing me as they changed the sheets and tried to stanch the blood flow.

Perhaps I'd already gained a mother's heightened sense of hearing, because at some point during that blur of time, the faint sound of a whimper roused me out of a groggy half sleep. I was surprised to see Ed, his head bowed and shoulders shaking, sitting by the window.

That Ed might be breaking down frightened me. I managed to mumble, "Ed, really, I'll be okay, please . . ."

By morning, I was finally alert enough to understand that Matt would likely be kept from me for the next forty-eight hours, the time it would take for the antibiotics to take effect and bring down my temperature. I first pleaded with, and then screamed at, every doctor that entered my room until one, a woman, yelled right back at me, "THE MEDICATION WILL WORK. YOU JUST HAVE TO WAIT. NOW STOP IT."

———

Two days later, upon seeing a nurse at my door with Matt in her arms, I practically choked on my excitement as both a sob and a laugh caught in my throat. I leaned forward (the pain shooting through my abdomen barely registered) and trembled as Matt was nestled into the crooks of my arms.

I was incredulous when the nurse then asked if the six nursing students now standing at the foot of my bed could watch me nurse for the first time. After two days of bottle-feeding, Matt might reject my breast; now I would have an audience to my second failure? But the teacher in me said yes, and ultimately I appreciated their delighted reaction when I nuzzled my nipple near Matt's mouth and Matt latched on hungrily. I finally felt like a mother.

———

It took me a few weeks to regain my energy as I recuperated from the surgery and blood loss while nursing a voracious infant. Sharing a weakness when it comes to long-term planning, Ed and I hadn't decided how and under what circumstances I would return to work. We had postponed the decision, hoping it would become clear once I had the baby.

Instead, Matt's arrival just exacerbated my conflict. I told myself (and others) that as a feminist, I didn't want to sacrifice my career and our financial situation by staying home, yet I suspected, privately, that I needed the feelings of self-esteem that practicing law afforded me—if only as seen through the eyes of others. At the same time, the idea that I might be selfish and heartless enough to risk harming Matthew's emotional development by returning to work was devastating to me.

My conflict was resolved when, less than a month after Matt's birth, Ed broke the news that due to issues at his new law firm, our financial situation was now, and for the foreseeable future, perilous. With a new mortgage to carry, I felt obligated to pursue a government job I'd recently heard about—law secretary to a judge—that offered a good salary, regular paychecks, and benefits. And so I returned to full-time work eleven weeks to the day after Matt was born.

To assuage my guilt and despite our pediatrician's serious doubts, I vowed to continue nursing Matt, no matter how difficult that might become.

———

I persuaded myself that a job that involved no clients, just research and drafting opinions, could not be as anxiety provoking as the job in the Riverhead practice. But I was soon proved wrong. The judge I was working for had an explosive temper, and though I'd gained some confidence as a mother, it hadn't translated to me as a lawyer. Like most new mothers, I was exhausted. My anxiety and fatigue were in some form of homeostasis—increased anxiety wired me awake while fatigue dulled the impact on my nerves.

Ten months later, when Ed's income became stable enough to meet our expenses, I was thrilled to quit that job.

———

About six months later, a friend, who also had a one-year-old, asked me to be her partner in a new clothing store, a commitment that would be part-time, seasonal, and, as we respected each other's maternal priorities, very flexible. Already somewhat bored with the ceaseless cycle of baby and household chores, I was excited to try something new. Ed and I were nervous about the financial risk involved, but the situation carried none of the anxiety familiar to me as a lawyer. It's possible I'd internalized the lopsided values of my father, who, prizing academic, intellectual, and professional endeavors above all else, practically disdained the strictly commercial. If running a business had no real value, then by some subconscious syllogism, my possible failure at it posed no emotional threat.

I didn't miss the intellectual aspects of practicing law and even enjoyed the repetitive tasks of processing inventory; I told one lawyer friend that I'd rather count Calvins than worry about losing a case.

But when I became pregnant with our second child, I decided to leave the store as soon after his birth as possible. Still guilt-ridden over the circumstances of Matt's early infancy— our almost three-day separation following his birth, then my return to work less than three months later—I was determined not to subject Peter, or me, to that trauma.

———

Fortunately for all of us, Peter's birth was a relatively easy one. Like Matt, he was two weeks late, but Peter, in what would become a defining characteristic of his personality, insisted on making his presence known. Thus, with my second son, labor started naturally, and although I couldn't avoid a C-section, his birth and my recovery were much more comfortable.

I took pleasure in watching our boys develop, and in our many games and routines. But I couldn't deny that on many days, I might as well have been slogging through mud, and even the simple task of emptying the dishwasher filled me with a kind of existential dread. At that point I refused to call it a depression—I was not my father, I reassured myself—but the heaviness I felt was undeniable and certainly impacting my kids. Terrified of recreating the conditions of my childhood, I returned to therapy.

I went back to work around the time Peter turned one, if only because I could no longer justify seeing my therapist, Barbara, without earning money to pay for the sessions. This time, however, I was determined to find a law job where I wasn't racked with anxiety and self-doubt.

I met with the senior partner of the Riverhead firm where I'd worked previously and negotiated the terms of a job that I hoped I could handle. I would work three days per week and specialize in wills and estates, a practice where the deadlines were predictable and the clients technically dead.

So far, my legal career had been nothing more than a gradual retreat from pressure. I hoped no one noticed as I slowly tiptoed backward from full-time associate at a large, high-powered New York City law firm to full-time associate at a small-town but high-powered law firm to a nine-to-five government law secretary job (which the rest of the profession considers part-time) to, finally, a part-time law job that one partner described as "lite law."

Ed was infinitely patient with my career contraction. He

just wanted me to be happy in my job. But even after all my changes, I had no idea what that meant. I knew what it meant to get through a day, to survive a week, to have a fleeting moment of pride before the next inevitable wave of anxiety hit. For the most part, every decision I made took on the gravity of life and death—or at least as close as a lawyer could get to that without actually stepping out onto a ledge. At every turn, and in spite of successes, I was haunted by the possibility that I would finally be exposed as the poseur I considered myself to be.

———

In 1994, when Matt and Peter were about eight and five respectively, we took a family hike in the White Mountains. Each day we would hike from peak to peak, and each night we'd stop at a cabin where good-natured college students would cook us dinner and assign us our bunk beds.

Peter seemed to fly over the rocks; close to the ground, he could maintain his balance over the trickier terrain. Matt ran ahead as well, but he was always the one to stop to point out an unusual lichen or feathery plant that had managed to survive above the tree line.

One afternoon, the sky took on a greenish-black cast and gusts of wind swirled unpredictably. We were fortunate to be a short walk from the tourist center at the top of Mount Washington; within minutes of our arrival, the center's anemometer registered 122 miles per hour. An announcement came over the sound system: *It is too dangerous to leave the building until further notice.*

When the wind had died down to about fifty miles per hour

and the rain had let up to a drizzle, we started out on a one-hour hike to the cabin where we'd be spending the night. Not having rain gear, we fashioned ponchos out of large black garbage bags distributed by the center's employees before setting off.

Ordinarily the trail was not dangerous. Although it snaked along the mountain's edge, there was a buffer of rocks about ten feet wide. But wind blowing at fifty miles per hour is loud enough to suck up words as soon as they're spoken—and strong enough to overpower a child. With no ballast against the wind, Peter's garbage bag became a sail, and he was soon all but airborne. Ed, who was ahead with Matthew, could not hear me screaming, "Ed, get Peter! He's going to go off the cliff! Get him!"

I was running after Peter, but with the wind in my face I made little headway. Peter was swept in Ed's direction, thank God, and no harm came to him.

With a happy ending, we could turn the incident into a fun family joke—but when I got home after this trip, I was so exhausted I could barely drag myself out of bed. Although I had found the hiking strenuous (I wasn't in the best physical shape), and got little sleep over the four nights we spent in a bunkroom with strangers, the source of my fatigue felt to me like something more than just physical depletion.

After a week I had more energy, but not the kind that makes you want to face a day. Although I forced myself to go to work, just the thought of it felt too heavy for my head. As I had said to my therapist at many other times, I felt like I was thigh deep in sludge and trying to walk through it.

My usual tactics of white knuckles, clenched jaw, and shoulders tensed for a struggle weren't working. After putting the kids to bed one night, I looked across the table at Ed and said, "I think I'm depressed. I just have this heavy feeling, like I'm fighting a sob all the time. It's too much effort to even think. I don't know if I can do this job, or *anything*, anymore."

"You should tell Barbara how bad it is."

"She knows." I wanted to ask Ed's opinion on something, but it was dangerous territory; it was important to me that his answer be "no." So I assumed a lighter tone, dragged myself out of the sludge for a moment, even managed a chuckle. "You don't think I need medication, do you? I guess a lot of people are taking stuff, but I'm not that bad. I'm sure I don't need it."

"Ame, I think you do. You should talk to Barbara about it."

"Are you serious?" I was sure he would say that it would pass like it had before—that I would snap out of it, that I couldn't be bad off enough for medication. To me, medication was one step away from hospitalization. I could picture the plastic, amber-colored vials in the cabinet in my parents' bathroom, their white labels bearing unpronounceable names and, along the top, "Harold M. Turner."

————

At my next session I asked Barbara what she thought of Ed's response to my question about medication. I chuckled then too, confident that she would dismiss it as an overreaction, completely inapplicable to the emotionally stable lawyer I pretended to be.

"You know," she said, "I agree. It's a good idea. Let me give you the name of a psychiatrist you can talk to about it."

My face flushed. She might as well have said that next she'd fit me for a straitjacket. "Really? I mean, I'm not that bad. I'm not crazy. I'm still working."

"I think it would help. It doesn't have to be this hard."

If I'd learned anything else from my father, it was to follow the advice of professionals you trust. So I did.

———

After a few tries, I found a medication that took the bottom out, that placed a floor above the abyss. Although decisions could still have serious consequences, they were no longer deadly. Still, I always mentioned to anyone who found out that it was a very low dose. "'Subclinical,' the shrink says. 'Probably not even therapeutic.' I guess I don't need much."

In other words, I was taking an antidepressant, but I *was not sick.*

———

Years later, I asked Barbara why she hadn't recommended medication sooner.

"Too dangerous for you, Amy," she said. "Your psyche was too fragile. If I'd suggested medication, you would have concluded you were seriously mentally ill, like your father had been. I'm not sure what would have happened to you then. I didn't want to risk it."

I recalled that when my father had told me he'd dropped or possibly flunked out of law school, I had seen the same fate for myself—a reflexive and lifelong sense that his failures had to be mine as well.

11

HAROLD AND HIS
PURPLE CRAYON

IN SEPTEMBER OF 2010, TWO MONTHS AFTER THE
accident and a week before I was to return to teaching, Ed and I
drove up to Vermont to visit Peter at college. We stopped at
Whole Foods on the way and sat down outside to eat the tofu-
this-and-that and other dishes we'd selected from the prepared
food bars. We were talking about plans for the weekend—where
to take Peter to dinner; which, if any, of the parents' weekend
activities we'd want to attend—when my cell phone rang.

I looked down and saw my brother Jim's number in Iowa.
Not wanting to talk on my cell in a public place, I sent his call to
voice mail and retrieved the message from there.

"Ame . . . It's Jim . . . Call me as soon as you can. Umm, it's
important."

I looked at Ed and shook my head slowly. After thirty years
of marriage, he knew my family as well as any of us knew each
other. "Harold?"

"It has to be. Oh God, I can't face it, not now."

We didn't talk as we finished eating. I savored the silence,
hung on to my final few minutes of ignorance, and felt grateful
my parents, having passed away years earlier, had been spared
this loss.

Sitting beside Ed in our parked car, I returned the call to learn what I already knew: Harold was dead.

For our own and each other's sakes, Jim and I tried hard to get through the call without tears, but it was difficult. Jim had had it much worse than I had in dealing with Harold. As the younger brother, Jim had been genetically wired to admire Harold but had also been his most readily available victim. For the previous fifteen years, the two of them had both lived in the same small town of Fairfield—where, I imagined, it had been almost impossible for Jim to shield himself from the consequences, emotional and otherwise, of Harold's drinking. Although he was too private a person to have ever shared his feelings with me, I was sure that when it came to dealing with Harold, Jim's burdens must have been far heavier and his emotions much more complex than mine.

When Jim described the policeman coming to his door and asking, "Are you the brother of Harold Turner? I'm sorry to inform you . . ." I could feel the threads that I thought had frayed to nothing long ago tighten around me in a final, fleeting hug, then snap one by one.

———

If I'd heard this news at any other time in the previous twenty years, I would have been sad but not surprised. Harold and his girlfriend (soon-to-be wife) had moved to Fairfield in 1987 or so—about a year after the birth of their daughter, Katherine— believing it would be the best environment in which to raise a child and perhaps for Harold to maintain sobriety.

Fairfield is not your typical small town in Iowa; even a quick glance at its downtown, with its several Indian restaurants and shops selling Ayurvedic products, Indian clothing, and gems recommended according to Vedic principles, indicates that something out of the Iowa ordinary is at work. And that would be the town's university, which occupies the site the former Parsons College—which thrived during the Vietnam War years due to offering college draft deferments to high school graduates whose only qualifications were being able to pay the enormous tuition—once did.

When Parsons closed in the seventies as the Vietnam War ended, the TM movement bought the campus and transformed it into the Maharishi University of Management (now called Maharishi International University), TM's centerpiece in the US. Eventually, it included two domed buildings in which, at times, thousands of men and women met to meditate twice a day.

TM and the therapeutic influence of thousands of meditators may have kept Harold alive for that period, but it couldn't eliminate his problem.

Eventually he was drinking too much to live with his wife, their daughter, and his wife's two sons. He moved from apartments to motels (which my mother financed for a while), and then alternated between the streets and the couches of bar acquaintances just slightly less down-and-out than he. By 1996, he was married to Trudy. "She's really nice, Ame, you would like her," he'd occasionally slur on my answering machine. But less than two years later, he was compelled to identify her body: she'd been murdered on her way home from a bar.

Arrested numerous times for public consumption of alcohol and vagrancy, for years Harold had called only to ask for money—initially polite requests that always ended in angry demands. And I still remembered how my head had pounded in rhythm with the percussive and frightening sounds of the hard *c*'s—"may not *recover* normal *cognitive* function, brain damage due to *continuous* grand mal seizures and *stroke, complications* from atypi*cal* psy*chotic* episodes, possibly electro*shock* therapy"—as a psychiatrist described Harold's condition eight years earlier, in 2002. Harold would recover well enough to eventually resume drinking.

But recently he had made amazing progress. He'd been off anti-seizure medication, cigarettes, coffee, and alcohol for the last three years, ever since his incarceration in an Iowa jail for public intoxication.

The turnaround had begun when, as he was being transported from the intake prison, which had an attached medical clinic, to a more restrictive facility, he'd experienced a major seizure. According to Jean, a smart, attractive, and relentlessly determined fifty-year-old woman whose relationship to Harold was, depending on one's point of view, girlfriend, guardian, or manipulator, she'd convinced the warden that moving Harold to a jail without a medical wing would constitute reckless endangerment at minimum. Apparently, the intake prison had offered two other advantages as well: it was more protective of inmates and prohibited smoking, which Jean considered a precursor to Harold's drinking. And so Harold had served out his eleven-month term (imposed because of his repeat offenses) in that facility, where Jean also persuaded the warden to give Harold juice and reading glasses.

Upon his release after almost a year of clean, healthy living, Harold, who'd rarely questioned Jean's plans for him, had proceeded to accomplish what he hadn't since he was in his twenties: just over a thousand consecutive days of being clean.

But because Harold still had memory lapses stemming from his prior alcohol abuse and stroke, he would occasionally forget who Jean was, let alone be grateful for what she did for him. At first about once a week, and less frequently as his memory improved, I'd come home to hear a message from him on my answering machine: "Umm, Ame, I'm out here with this woman, Jean. I don't think you know her. She's pretty and all, but she's such a pain in the ass. I can't drink or smoke or even have a cup of coffee. She's living here or something and is such a bitch." (I would have been alarmed by this message if there hadn't also been signs that Harold's memory was otherwise improving.) And then his voice would trail off, and he'd continue on to another topic that reflected his confusion: "I saw someone today and I told them I am so lucky. I have the sexiest, smartest, prettiest sisters in the world, and they live in New York and are so cool . . ."

Mercifully, the machine would cut him off before he moved on to another delusion.

Although I'd been grateful to Jean for her dedication to Harold, I hadn't fully understood it until she explained that years earlier, she and Harold had visited a jyotishi (Vedic astrologer) who read their birth charts. According to his chart, Harold's life would burn intensely, leading him down a path to either spiritual bliss or hellish torment. The jyotishi had told Jean that she was in the presence of a "pious man with a pure heart" and that she should take care of him.

In 2008, when I'd last seen Harold, the proof of his sobriety had been obvious. He had started using his right arm again (which had been severely limited due to his stroke), his memory had improved, and his face had a faint pink glow rather than the corpse-like pallor of an alcoholic.

At lunch in a Fairfield restaurant, I'd looked across the table at my brothers and recalled why, as a child, I'd begun to think that of the three of us, Harold might be the most special. In one of my parents' few joint expressions of playfulness (which my sister apparently originated), we were each accorded a song that featured our first names. Although "Once in Love with Amy" mostly embarrassed me, I loved it when my parents referred to the song or, in my father's case, sang a few lines from it. For a child like me, it offered tangible proof that our family was inseparably bound to each other, if only by having names distinctive enough to appear in a song.

Although Harold's song—"Hark the Herald Angels Sing"— was a bit of a stretch, he also had what our family prized above all—a book, actually a series of books, with his name in the title: *Harold and the Purple Crayon*. Published in 1955, a year after Harold's birth, it had been ready for him just as he was ready to be read to. Fictional Harold, about four years old and appearing simply as a black outline on a background of white, could realize all his dreams and escape all perils, even those he created, by drawing one unbroken line with his large purple crayon. He drew himself to the moon and escaped a dragon and a near drowning, and however far away his adventures took him, in the end he always remembered how to draw himself back to where he most wanted to be: at home, sleeping in his own bed, the blanket literally drawn up to his chin, his face at peace under a moon perfectly framed in his window.

When Harold told stories from his college days during that lunch with Jim and me, his joy cast a soft focus on him so that I could no longer make out his receding hairline or the canyons that years of drinking had carved into his face. As children, Harold, Jimmy, and I had all been platinum blondes, but Harold's hair darkened earlier and to a greater degree than ours. In the summer, his light brown freckles gained territory and could almost masquerade as a tan. Invariably, his face would also have red patches where the freckles stopped and the zinc oxide had been hastily applied, if at all.

Even when his hair was darker, the sun would still bleach the tips of his eyelashes silver, and depending on his clothing or his mood, Harold's eyes could shift from blue to hazel to green. Later on, whenever the whites of his eyes looked a little yellow or murky, he would claim that it was evidence of digestive complications resulting from an imbalance in his colon, surely not related to his heavy drinking.

One could say that Harold's nose was too thick—a little unrefined, perhaps, for the patrician life my parents had envisioned for him. But it was straight and without bulges or bumps, and remained that way despite the bar fights. Harold also had a broad smile and wasn't self-conscious about his teeth, despite their yellowish cast. The gap between his two front teeth refused to close, giving him a look, as he got older, of boyishness and a certain roguishness.

When Jim was old enough to parrot whatever I said, we gave Harold the nickname Head. It was not, of course, a prediction of his future pot use, but rather a literal reference to his inordinately large head. It bobbled, as if too heavy for his trunk. Perhaps I made fun of him out of envy, already sensing that this malformation might be the price he'd have to pay for having a brain far more talented than mine. But by eighteen, Harold's Mr. Potato

Head–like head was the appropriate size for his slim six-foot-two frame, and any imperfections in his face either disappeared or melded into an undeniable, if unconventional, handsomeness. His once gangly arms and legs also found proportion, making him a natural for dancing, tennis, and basketball—any activity that required a glide. The images of him in effortless motion are what stay with me: on the dance floor at my wedding, moving with an innate rhythm that belied our physically uptight upbringing; on a tennis court, arcing fluidly through a forehand; and on a basketball court, launching the ball toward the basket with one graceful flick of his palms and fingertips, his body erect, suspended two feet in the air. It was impossible even for me, his sister, to ignore that above all else, Harold was sexy. And that would save him on more than one occasion.

———

A week before Harold's memorial service, I started to think about what I might say at the event. For inspiration, I began an archaeological dig in our basement to locate a box of my old letters. After about a half hour of trying to avoid inhaling mildew as I unstacked and restacked cardboard boxes, I finally found it. The pink stationery of our high school English teacher Patsy Ribner—her letters to me during 1971 and 1972, my school year in Switzerland—was easy to spot. Desperately wanting one more time to be an eighteen-year-old girl with a seventeen-year-old brother, I sat on the basement floor and, as the tears streaked the dust on my face, read them all.

Had I taken the letters upstairs to read, the dig would have ended there, and I never would have noticed in the corner oppo-

site me an unfamiliar trunk that served as foundation for a sky-
scraper of boxes. I quickly removed each box to reveal the kind
of trunk we had taken to summer camp—its once shiny black
surface peeling and gray, its reinforced corners dented, and its
metal lock now rusted and disintegrating. When I opened it, I
felt I may as well have been peering into Harold's coffin, because
there he was, documented in report cards, newspaper clippings,
academic awards, childhood drawings, college essays, and post-
cards from camp.

Also in the trunk, in a stack held together by a deteriorating
rubber band, were my letters to him. When I unfolded the light
blue tissue aerogram and saw my rounded, girlish print, I was
embarrassed for my eighteen-year-old self who had thought her
naive threats—"Mom's going to kill you if you don't stop doing
drugs"—could solve Harold's problem, but also realized she had
not yet been jaded by the decades of worry and unheeded pleas
that would follow.

I examined each artifact, hoping that this autopsy of sorts
might reveal the source of his suffering. There was the expected
anatomy of any talented and privileged man—glowing report
cards, newspaper clippings of undefeated basketball seasons,
trophies won in county tennis tournaments, academic awards,
and childhood drawings. There were the cards for Christmas
and Mother's Day and Father's Day, the products of obligatory
elementary school activities, but then there were others that I
am certain no schoolteacher had a hand in: Harold had written
thank-you notes to our parents that as a child I would never have
written, or as a parent could never have expected to receive.
There were notes thanking them for Christmas presents, a trip
to a football game, for a special trumpet, for just being "great

parents," to name a few. Although I could still picture Harold on a tennis court as a child—zinc-oxided nose, straw-blond hair, and slightly sunburned face, fighting back tears whenever he lost to his best friend, whose only advantage was a killer instinct—I hadn't remembered him as particularly sensitive. His anger and arrogance, the by-products of decades of drinking, had obliterated most of my memories of his vulnerability and sweetness. But as I read a note he'd written at age ten to my parents, "Thank you very much for making Sat. the 25th such a wonderful day, someday I'll do it for you . . ." and one he'd written eight years later to my father regarding their victory in a crucial doubles match, "Perhaps the time that has passed since our glorious match has wrapped our experience in gold. Whatever the case may be, gold or fool's gold, I will treasure it the same," all echoes of those drunken rants were gone, and in the silence I could almost hear the soft beating of his heart.

———

A few nights before I left for the funeral, Jean was eager to tell me how Harold had died, as she considered the circumstances of the kind that holy people might pray for and a clear sign that Harold was an extraordinary person. The day before, Harold had refused his favorite Indian lunch for the first time ever and eaten nothing thereafter. (In Jean's view, Harold had intuitively followed the Vedic prescription that advises against eating within twenty-four hours before death.) That night he'd told Jean that he'd just had two great telephone conversations: one with his daughter, Katherine, and the other with Jim, who had told him to "hold fast." Jean had been so happy that Harold had had a

chance on the same day to speak to the two people most important to him—but when she checked his cell phone, she saw that
no calls had been made or received.

The next morning Jean had left early for group meditation,
after first making sure that Harold was warmly covered in bed.
When she returned three hours later, she'd found him on the
floor. As she described how the duvet had been draped over his
body (in a way that suggested to her a traditional Vedic crema-
tion ceremony), I envisioned him in a cocoon of white comforter—its edges almost carefully, and perhaps lovingly, tucked
under his chin to reveal only his face.

After hearing the story, I couldn't quite console myself with
a belief in Harold's piety and purity, but I was relieved for him,
and for us even more so, that he'd died peacefully, of "natural
causes." Had he died at many other times in his life, there would
surely have been painful details—bar fights, street living, drinking, drugs, jail—which would have eliminated the possibility of
comforting ourselves with a story of his redemption.

Soon after my call with Jean, I spoke to Harold's twenty-
four-year-old daughter, Katherine, about the funeral service.
When she said she planned to share a "children's book" that
meant a great deal to both of them, I knew its title before she
mentioned it. But I was surprised (and touched) to learn that
Harold had often read *Harold and the Purple Crayon* to her over
the phone as an adult, even so recently as last month. Harold
had never stopped creating his own perils, yet he must have
hoped that one day, like the fictional Harold, he would be able
to draw his means of escape and find himself at home, at peace,
safe from himself. He had finally done just that.

———

Although I was comforted by what Jean told me about Harold's death, and by the prospect of listening to Katherine read *Harold and the Purple Crayon*, I needed a lot of steady support at Harold's funeral. Three months after the accident, I still had little tolerance for noise, chatter, or speed. I told Ed that I was just uncomfortable, too embarrassed to admit that I had trouble keeping up. But Ed couldn't take the time off to accompany me to Fairfield, and frankly, I felt he'd already done enough for me where my family was concerned. Peter was busy at college, but Matt agreed to come with me.

Although Matt, at twenty-four, could often be distracted, he must have noticed me taking more than the few seconds necessary to locate our flight on the departures screen and decided that I would not be a reliable navigator, because he quickly took charge at the airport, leading me through the maze of airport ticketing and security at LaGuardia and then on the dash through O'Hare to find our connection to Cedar Rapids, Iowa.

By the time we landed in Iowa, there was no question that Matt would be the driver on our ninety-minute trip to Fairfield. As we left the airport, I had to shake the sensation that we'd landed in another universe. Just hours earlier, we'd been driving to a New York airport on a crowded six-lane highway that seemed to disappear into a concrete sky. And now, stretching to the horizon, was an almost empty road, on either side an expanse of deep-green soybean fields dotted by a smattering of farmhouses and barns.

After we settled into our rented car, Matt let me choose the radio station. I was lazily turning the dial through snippets of static, evangelical sermons, and country music when my fingers jerked to a stop—even before I fully recognized the familiar notes of "The Logical Song."

"Oh God, Matthew, this is one of Harold's favorite songs. I cannot believe we are hearing it now. I can picture him singing it. We were coming home from college together. He was driving, sitting next to me, just like you are."

I lifted the lever along the side of my seat and pressed my head back. As the seat reclined, I closed my eyes. I could never have predicted that a truck would hit me in a crosswalk or that Harold would die when he had seemed healthier than he'd been in years. I had been determined to get back to work, to return to normal, to move forward as quickly as possible and forget that I'd been injured. But Harold's death was pulling me in the opposite direction. Instead of preparing for my return to work, I was revisiting my distant past and feelings I'd either forgotten or long ago dismissed. Years later, I would wonder if the primal connection we'd shared had less to do with our being thirteen months apart than it had with our seeking the sense of security that in those early years our alcoholic mother and suicidal father could not provide.

I felt that the song was Harold's message to me, that we'd been forgiven, that whatever pain we'd caused each other—his drinking, my inability, and at times unwillingness, to help him— could no longer obscure what we'd felt since his birth: a bond that, had we known the word for it back then, would have been love.

12

ISABELLA

THREE MONTHS AFTER BEING HIT BY A TRUCK AND two days after attending my brother's funeral, returning to teach seventh graders six weeks into the school year was more disorienting than suddenly being thrust into the middle of a competitive tennis match in progress. As I sat in front of my first class (my doctor recommended that I stay off my feet as much as possible), I thought my dizziness was causing the slight tremor in the room. But I'd forgotten the collective power of eleven- and twelve-year-olds. Even when they are perfectly silent and still, any seasoned middle school teacher can feel their energy hum.

The best way for me to readjust was to start my classes the way I always did in September—by asking the students why we study history. After we finished discussing "so as not to repeat the mistakes of the past," I wrote a new reason to study history on the whiteboard: "It really helps when you are hit by a truck."

The students' chatter stopped immediately, but I knew from their puzzled expressions that they wanted to ask a question.

"Yes," I said, "I'm serious. It really helped me." As I told the story (without graphic details), I realized that for them the most preposterous part of my story was not that I had stood in a crosswalk and watched a truck barrel into me but that I had actually blabbered about George Washington as I lay on the sidewalk and the Vietnam War as I had been hoisted into a helicopter.

"Really, Ms. Turner, you said that? You did not . . . You're joking. Nobody does that . . . Really?" they asked incredulously.

I don't know whether I convinced them that history could help them to overcome future challenges, but their close-to-perfect behavior that first week suggested that they had learned something else: don't even try to mess with a teacher who's stared down an oncoming truck.

And so my students were the easy part about returning to work—but the teaching routines were not. I was too dizzy to move my head, which ached more than usual when I was compelled to explain that Martin Luther King Jr. did not free the slaves, and writing on the board aggravated my shoulder injury. After two classes, my scapula burned so much that it hurt to stand up straight, so I stooped slightly to my left, dangling my arm like a broken wing.

Dr. Friedman suggested I see an acupuncturist.

———

I was well aware of acupuncture's value. A few years before the accident, Ed and I had seen Dr. Pai, a practitioner in New York City.

We had learned about Dr. Pai from Ed's younger brother, Paul, who had married Kelley, a recently licensed acupuncturist. When Kelley learned that Ed had been struggling with Lyme disease and taking buckets of antibiotics for almost two years, she motivated Ed (or, as he would say, relentlessly badgered him) into consulting her acupuncture professor in New York City. Dr. Pai was also a leading authority on Chinese herbs and had a specialty in psychiatry as practiced in traditional Chinese medicine. When I developed a swimming overuse injury in 2007, I was grateful that Dr. Pai was already in our lives, and very soon I was seeing him weekly.

At the beginning of each visit, Dr. Pai would speak with me in his office for twenty minutes while he made his assessment and prescribed herbs. Then I would go into the treatment room and lie on a bed as he "needled" me. While I remained on the treatment table for twenty minutes in a near meditative state, Dr. Pai would meet with Ed, then come back and remove my needles. Dr. Pai's protocol ran like clockwork, but there was nothing mechanical about his style. His warmth and humor were always evident.

At the end of one visit, I recalled now, Dr. Pai had offered a slight shake of his head and a half smile, and announced, "Oh, I wish I could plant your feet and unchain your mind!" I understood what he meant by the first part—he'd frequently urged me to get more rest, drink less coffee . . . just slow down. But I asked him to explain "unchaining my mind." Whether he didn't answer because of the limitations of his English, his generally laconic nature, or the lack of talk therapy in traditional Chinese medicine's version of psychiatry, I couldn't be sure.

Dr. Pai had likely sensed back then what I could barely admit to myself—that a part of me was inaccessible, frozen in contraction, like some impossible-to-reach muscle that refused to let go. Decades of meditation and therapy and a year of acupuncture with Dr. Pai had not yet unclenched it, and that realization both scared and shamed me. I couldn't shake the sensation that, despite all my efforts, on the deepest level, something was wrong with me.

For years I had kept this from Ed, who occasionally asked,

most often after intimate encounters, whether I might be holding something back. Each time, I vehemently objected. I needed to reassure myself that I'd done the work. I understood myself. I was not sick.

I recalled the times I'd seen iron bars in my mind, just as I felt the downward tug of a dark mood. As absurd to me as it had seemed even then, I'd tried each time to squeeze through the prison door by thinking uplifting thoughts, or picturing open fields, or using any other mental powers I could muster. It had rarely worked.

I was simultaneously the guard and the prisoner, which made for a strange and endless feedback loop.

———

After the accident, I was in too much pain to manage a weekly five-hour round trip to and from Manhattan to see Dr. Pai, so Dr. Friedman recommended Isabella James, a local acupuncturist. He described her as fantastic but "a little outside the box." I didn't care how unusual her methods were, I just wanted the pain to stop.

Isabella lived and worked just a few minutes from my school, where every forty minutes a roiling mass of eleven- and twelve-year-olds shrieked and shoved and laughed their way down the hall to their next class; kindergartners, the "ankle biters," tried to stand quietly in neat lines but invariably found something to laugh at or someone to poke; and all of us had become inured to the harsh glare of fluorescent lights, the lingering smell of mold, and the dirt that was a permanent feature of the eighty-year-old building.

Yet what a difference a few minutes could make. The path to Isabella's home was shaded by a stand of evergreen trees and curved through knee-high plants, their foliage ranging from greenish black to light jade. A stone birdbath seemed to have grown up from a bed of pachysandra, and I had just noticed the smooth pale-colored pebbles in the lap of a seated Buddha statue when I heard the slight whine of a screen door.

Isabella stood in the entrance of the house, her right arm outstretched to hold the door open for me. Her hair, the color of dark chocolate, was pulled back from her face, which gleamed slightly, perhaps from the hint of gold in her complexion. She reminded me of the longtime meditators I'd seen in Fairfield, whose beauty never needed the distraction or amplification of makeup.

As soon as I walked through the door, I felt I'd entered a different dimension. The fragrances of essential oils, the teals and roses of the handmade quilts, the delicate details of the botanical watercolors, the careful rows of glass bottles, and the utter silence were so calming that I struggled to keep my eyes open as she asked me routine intake questions.

When she inquired about any prior experience with acupuncture, I replied that I had seen Dr. Pai in New York.

"Dr. Pai?" she repeated slowly, as though she hadn't quite heard me. She looked down and slowly shook her head, as if giving herself a few moments to absorb my words. Then she smiled, her liquid brown eyes sparkling. "He's my mentor—I've seen him once a month ever since I had him as a professor. I'm amazed. You're the first person I know out here who has even heard of him, let alone seen him."

"Oh my God," I said. "You can't believe what he's meant to me and my husband."

Isabella and I smiled at each other for longer than any two strangers would normally feel comfortable.

After repeating a few more times, "I can't believe it," Isabella invited me to lie down on the treatment table. As she stood over me, she sensed my tension. "Are you okay?"

"It's just that Dr. Pai . . ." I hesitated, afraid that what I was thinking might insult her. "I mean I loved him, and his treatments were great, but God, he could jab those needles in."

Isabella laughed. "Yes, I know. That is how he does it. But with you I had planned to use the finest-gauge needles, from France, actually. You should barely feel them."

My apprehension dissolved as Isabella smoothed an alcohol-soaked cotton ball in dime-sized circles on my ankles, wrists, and ears. Usually I wouldn't even have noticed this preliminary step, but Isabella's touch drew my attention as if she were inviting my body to join the healing process. The prick of the first needle was subtle, like the nip of an insect one doesn't bother to brush away. I barely flinched, and as I exhaled, my shoulders softened against the table.

All week, I looked forward to my next appointment. The serenity alone was the perfect antidote to the stresses of teaching. The combination of warm stone massage (Isabella was a licensed masseuse as well) and acupuncture calmed my shoulder spasm and allowed for greater mobility.

During one of my first visits, I asked Isabella about her diploma from Oberlin College. She said she'd focused on art and after college had lived in New York City, where she designed textiles. I was lying prone on the treatment table, at that point staring at the floor through the face cradle, the edges of which squeezed against my eyebrows and chin. Standing metal lamps were focused on my back, their beams radiating through gems selected for their healing properties. I mumbled a question about her change from art to acupuncture. She mentioned that she had been on a Metro North platform when she'd met the person who had encouraged her to make the switch.

At the end of her story, I said, still speaking to the floor, "Metro North. Were you in Westchester?"

"Yes, I was."

"Oh, whereabouts?"

"Bronxville."

I jerked my head up so I could gasp. "Did you grow up there?"

"Yes," she replied, dragging out the word, already seeming to intuit that something unusual was coming. I had already started to laugh. During my thirty years in East Hampton, I had met only one other year-round resident originally from Bronxville. As Isabella appeared to be in her forties, at least fifteen years younger than me, it was not at all surprising that we hadn't known each other in Bronxville.

At that point I could have asked her anything: when she had lived there, whether we had known any of the same families or lived anywhere near each other. But my next questions came without thought, as though my brain had been tapped with a reflex hammer.

"Did you go to Bronxville High School?"

"Yes."

"Did you have Patsy Ribner?"

"Yes." I could hear the laughter in her voice as she spoke even faster. "She was my English teacher, SAT tutor. She helped me with my college application. And she's the one who taught me how to write."

I sat up suddenly, raising my voice over the sound of the lamps clattering to the floor that I'd forgotten had been trained on my back. "Oh, Jesus—she taught *me* how to write—she was my favorite teacher—I still have a paper that she corrected over forty years ago . . ."

Isabella smiled at me again, clearly as surprised as I was. We exchanged phrases of disbelief as I worked my way back to the chair at her desk. Almost as an afterthought, I asked what she'd written about for that college application essay.

"I suppose my topic was a little unusual. But it was on *Alice in Wonderland.*"

I looked up from the check I'd been writing. I could tell Isabella was anticipating another connection. I shrugged my shoulders and offered my open palms as if to say, "What gives?"

"That paper I wrote for Patsy that's still in my basement? That was about *Alice in Wonderland* too."

Isabella closed her eyes for a second and smiled. I asked her why she had chosen *Alice.*

"Oh, that's an easy one. It was the magic!"

I laughed to myself. *I should have known.* I'd already experienced a hint of magic in her office. I wondered if I might experience transformation as well.

––––

Isabella later suggested that I write about the accident, but I had already covered that ground with Barbara, my therapist. I imagined Barbara thought writing would serve as a prophylactic against PTSD, but I couldn't write about the accident. Not yet. When she gently probed my resistance, I heard an iron door clank, and like a petulant toddler I had access to only one word: "No."

Whenever I thought about writing, the feeling that I needed to know the end of the story before I could begin overwhelmed me. But I had no idea what I meant by "the end." Eventually I told Barbara that I might be afraid that my physical injuries would worsen and I didn't want to write about, let alone live with, prolonged pain or illness. I confessed to a superstition that writing about the accident might invite into my life a series of even more disturbing events. After all, Harold had died unexpectedly less than three months after I'd been hit by the truck. What might come next?

Although those explanations may have partially explained my resistance, I knew at the time they weren't the all of it; I didn't feel the relief that comes from an authentic confession.

It would be years before I'd recognize the truth: I'd been afraid that in writing about the accident, I might uncover in the experience of writing something more profound and more painful than physical injuries—and I wasn't ready for that.

13

WRITING

WRITING, FOR ME, HAD ALWAYS BEEN TREACHEROUS ground. After all, it seemed to be the cause of—or, alternatively, a major symptom of—my father's psychiatric problems. Although he never discussed his writing blocks, he might as well have broadcast them through the darkening black crescents under his eyes and his glassy, blank stare. He was not much of an advertisement for the endeavor. More than difficult, writing appeared to be dangerous.

Yet as children, my siblings and I valued that activity above all else. After all, it was our father's lifelong goal to be recognized as a writer, most preferably by *The New Yorker*. And so from the beginning, I, too, wanted to be a writer, either to gain my father's approval or perhaps to compensate for his failures. But I could never escape the dread that descended each time I picked up a pen or sat at the typewriter. If I got myself to produce more than a few words, invariably I'd find that "Turner sludge," that quicksand of sadness, swallowing even the lightest of stories.

For years, my father wrote at his heavy mahogany desk, installed in the bedroom he shared with my mother at 35 Valley, with the soft number one pencils he sharpened with a penknife. I could always trace his whereabouts or the progress of his writing by examining the yellow-tinged shavings. The trail would tell you where he'd been; the volume would tell you the amount he'd written. The larger the pile, the fewer words drafted. Instead of writing, he had been whittling the lead, engaged in a losing battle with his persistent writer's block.

Eventually the pile of pencil lead dust under his desk began to resemble a city built by industrious ants, and—whether due to the strain between my parents or my father's wishful thinking about the creative influence of a new location—he moved his work to a room located just off their bedroom. Soon suffering from writer's block again, he escaped by moving his work downstairs. That would be in my mother's territory, so it would be up to her whether to allow him to move his boxes of papers and towers of yellow legal pads filled with pages on which very few words survived his cross-outs, slashes that resembled flesh wounds more than pencil marks.

In the end she sequestered him to what we still called "the playroom," where, a decade before, Harold and Jimmy and I had spent rainy days sprawled on the toy-covered linoleum floor. Was she making a statement about his writing? It couldn't be denied that decades had passed and the only piece of his writing that had been published (in 1984) was an adaptation of his 1965 master's thesis for an introduction to the journals of John D'Wolf, Herman Melville's seafaring uncle. (Academic writing caused him no less turmoil than the more personal kind. In 1972 he earned a PhD in library science from New York University, an accomplishment of which we were all very proud. But it came only after years of struggle writing his dissertation—the name of his typist was as familiar to the family as his psychoanalyst— and, as my mother told it, her last-minute intervention. Emotionally distraught on the day of the final deadline, my father announced that his dissertation was such a failure it couldn't be submitted. Refusing to let him defeat himself, my mother somehow convinced him to get into the car and, after a forty-five-minute drive into NYC, hand-deliver the manuscript.)

But the small Rhode Island firm that published his master's thesis was not *The New Yorker*, which in our house was treated with reverential longing, as in my father's estimation it published the finest writing of the time. So, although every one of his submissions to *The New Yorker*—their topics as various as childhood memories, his experiences in Bangladesh, and his protest activities—had been politely rejected, my father gallantly soldiered on, now in the playroom, pencil in hand, penknife nearby.

Even while he was working on my mother's turf, the major form of communication between them was the notes they wrote in the spiral notebook located on the small yellow Formica table next to the stove in the kitchen. Whenever I came home from college, if I wanted a quick update on what had been going on, or the status of my parents' relationship, I would just leaf through its pages. Mom wrote with the blue BIC ballpoint that was always next to the pad. Dad wrote in his soft lead scrawl.

"Harold, playing tennis, getting hair done, and will leave some food for dinner."

"Virginia, going into NYC for dentist, Harold called, needs money. Happy anniversary, have a little gift for you. Want to go out to dinner tonight?"

"Harold, our anniversary is next month, not sure about dinner."

He would encourage all of his children to write, going as far in my case as to show the stories I'd written in a college creative writing class to a published author whom he knew. It was particularly generous of him, as a few of the stories portrayed him in a less-than-flattering light. I remember reading one of the stories to my college class; the professor remarked on my "attention to detail," and after a moment of stunned silence a student asked, "Did that really happen? Did he really give you a case of canned New England clam chowder for Christmas?" But for my father, his hurt feelings, if he had any, were of little concern. Writing was that important. "Just get it out, get it down," he used to say, "whatever it is."

I don't know if my father himself felt the sludge, but I could always detect it in his writing. In one case, what began as an affecting piece about a swim in a rough ocean during the summer of 1921 was hijacked later on by an episode of the darkest cruelty. In another piece, he wrote from the viewpoint of himself as a five-year-old, a moving story in which he portrayed a child's need for both wonder and love in touching and convincing detail. However, the sludge crept in about halfway through and by the end swallowed the piece whole: Harold and Jim, his sons, entered the story as adults whom he, the child, then pathetically begged to take care of him.

My father, proud of the piece, sent it to all of his children; we all, as I recall, had great difficulty disguising our aversion.

I always thought that my father's best writing appeared in his correspondence, both formal and casual, and in the personal recollections he recorded to entertain his children or grandchildren. Whenever my father managed to crawl out from under his self-imposed pressure to publish or sneak away from his internal editor, his writing hit the mark—blending the light and dark in perfect proportion. I particularly liked a remembrance that he had illustrated with two photographs of himself at about age four—one, captioned "Harold in repose," in which he wears a boater's hat with ribbon and the other, captioned "Harold at rest," in which his chin-length blond pageboy is unfettered—that said:

> Sundays in Chappaqua (and New York for a time
> when we moved there) there could be no games, no
> comic strips, no Maggie and Jiggs, no Mutt and Jeff, no
> Katzenjammer Kids. Nothing.
>   But some Sunday afternoons Dad did relent. One
> Sunday it was target practice with the family's .22, the
> target an empty sarsaparilla bottle mounted on a box.
>   Being older than I, Jack, Martha, and Rosamund
> shot ahead of me in that order, how well or poorly I
> haven't the faintest recollection.
>   When at last my turn came, Daniel Boone I was not.
> As I kept missing the bottle, until the muzzle of the .22
> was all but touching it, and at last I did hit it.
>   I remember Dad's comment, a little ambiguous I
> thought at the time and still do. "Very good, Harold," he
> said, "but very hard to miss." Maybe he was trying to get
> it across as delicately as he could that I was no Daniel
> Boone. No Davy Crockett either. Perhaps not even a
> straight shooter.

Of course, whatever the "genre," my father's writing never made *The New Yorker*'s cut. The rejection slips I found after his death at age ninety, in 2004, carefully filed in an unmarked manila folder, were poignant, to say the least.

A few years after discovering those slips, I started reading *Cheerful Money,* a memoir by Tad Friend, a staff writer for *The New Yorker.* I was interested because his family had been long-time members of the Georgica Association, where we spent our childhood summers and where I still belonged. I assumed my mother would be mentioned, since she had founded the association's tennis program and Tad and his family were avid tennis players, but there was absolutely no reason to expect a reference to my father—so when, about twenty-five pages after my mother's name came up, Tad mentioned my father, I yelled out so suddenly I wasn't even sure the sound had come from me. For a second it felt as if my father were sitting there in bed between Ed and me—a shocking prospect even if he hadn't been dead for five years.

My father's presence was that palpable because *his* were the words I was reading. According to Tad Friend, my father had written to Tad's grandfather, who was very ill at the time, to "say how much their conversations over the years had meant to him." My father's note read:

> There are very few people who are willing to give us a
> real listen, not strangers, certainly not acquaintances,
> not even good friends as a regular matter, not even
> *family* sometimes. But a good clubmate by virtue of the
> original nature of the experience will. He's been bred to
> it by the experience. And what, Dingleman, is more
> precious in this world than someone who will listen?

Of course, I can't know for sure how my father would have reacted to reading his note in that book. I'm sure the feelings would have been mixed. Although many of his Skull and Bones clubmates at Yale had been dear and devoted lifelong friends, over the years he'd become embarrassed by his membership in that elite enclave, and he might not have wanted to be quoted in that context. But I do think he would have considered, at least privately, the publication of his note as an affirmation, if only minimal, of his writing ability. Although he could not have missed the irony of Tad's association with *The New Yorker*, I wonder if he would have recognized another irony: it was a personal note to a friend—a piece of writing that would not have caught the attention of his internal critic or have attracted the Turner sludge—that ultimately saw print.

In any event, that occasion would be the closest he ever got to being published in *The New Yorker*, if only in a second-cousin-once-removed kind of way.

While my father never gave up his struggle to write, I abandoned the effort in my late twenties. It would be three decades before I wrote again, and by then, for reasons I don't fully understand but for which I'm grateful, it was not the Turner sludge I found but its antidote.

14

"STRENGTH IN WHAT
REMAINS BEHIND"

JIM HAD MENTIONED TO ME AT HAROLD'S FUNERAL
in Fairfield that he planned to organize a memorial service the
following spring in Bronxville, to give East Coast friends an opportunity to formally remember Harold.

About a month before the service, in May of 2011, Jim casually mentioned that the service had been moved from Bronxville
to St. Ann's in Bridgehampton, ten minutes from my house.
With that news, I had to cope with more than just grief: I
couldn't avoid offering to host a gathering afterward. And when
it became apparent that the gathering was going to be something of a high school reunion, I dreaded it even more.

For many, this would have been an inconvenience, but for Ed
and me, whose house was far too small for the number expected
and whose backyard looked like a brush dump, it would call for
heroics. With the help of two very generous friends and two local masons I hired out of desperation at the railroad station, we
transformed the visible part of our backyard into an acceptable,
if not beautiful, place for a garden party and screened the rest.

I was faced with transforming my house, teaching school,
and mourning my brother anew—all of which I might have been
able to handle if I were not also still dealing with the aftermath

of my accident. I still had to be very careful, as an overly intense shrug of my shoulder or a reach above my head to write on the blackboard was likely to cause spasms. My head still ached where it had hit the pavement, and any quick movement made me dizzy and off-balance. These injuries, along with the fatigue from the daily grind of teaching seventh graders, made each day more than the usual struggle. The rate at which those eleven- and twelve-year-olds asked questions reminded me of my mother's tennis Ball-Boy machine, which spit out tennis balls so quickly you could barely get your racket swung back before the next one bounced at your feet.

Before the accident, I could think fast enough to interrupt the barrage and redirect the questioner in a way that would promote reflection. But afterward, on many days, in pain and exhausted, I just let the questions fly by.

"Ms. Turner, what are we supposed to do here?"

"Read the directions."

"What?"

"Just read the directions."

"What? Where?"

"At the top of the page."

"Oh, I get it."

"Good. Let's get to work."

"Wait a minute, where are the directions? Oh, okay. It's about Hitler."

"Hey, Ms. Turner, why did he have that mustache?"

"Yeah, and anyway, why didn't they just call him 'Adolf'? Why do they always say 'Hitler'?"

And repeat, repeat, repeat—different students, different questions.

My weekly sessions with Isabella were a necessity if I wanted to do any more than crawl through the week. She used different methods—warm stone massage, acupressure, acupuncture, gem light therapy, and essential oils—and my confidence in her ran deep. On the concrete and superficial level, each treatment was gradually bringing improvement: lessening the severity of my headaches, reducing the frequency of my dizziness, and extracting the fatigue which seemed to have settled deep in my bone marrow. And on a more profound level, I was certain that the connections between us (growing up in Bronxville and our special connections to Patsy Ribner and Dr. Pai, to name only a few) meant she could help me in ways I couldn't yet foresee, or for that matter even understand.

After treatment, I usually came home with some amusing story for Ed. One afternoon, a fat white rabbit appeared in Isabella's neighborhood, and in the ensuing weeks it often showed up in her yard just before my appointment, which we attributed to our shared love of *Alice in Wonderland*. There were more than a few occasions when I'd mention to Isabella some random item, anything from a jade tree to a melon, and she'd smile and say, "Wait a minute," then retrieve the item I'd just mentioned, explaining that it had recently arrived in the mail or on her doorstep. These types of occurrences quickly became common enough that I began to expect them.

When the day of Harold's second memorial finally arrived, I was grateful for the beautiful weather and for the fact that my whole family was there, including my nieces, Laura and Katherine. It struck me that I was the matriarch that day (my sister, Louise, would not attend, as funerals had for her become too painful since the loss of her son)—and if I had doubted that I was old, all I had to do was look into the faces of the former classmates who attended.

During the service, memories of being in that same church—Harold, Jimmy, and I squirming next to our mother on summer Sunday mornings; my father walking me down the aisle; the entire family watching as water was sprinkled on the forehead of my nephew, Tom, now tragically deceased—floated back through time and grief, reuniting us all for a moment.

As much as I had dreaded this second memorial, I realized, sitting there, that it was a gift. It had brought the cousins, Matthew, Peter, Katherine, and Laura, together for the first time in more than twelve years, and their collective presence resurrected a meld of generations: Harold, brother, father, and uncle; Tom, nephew, brother, and cousin; and my parents, their grandparents.

As I looked at the cousins sitting next to each other in the church, I thought of the previous night. I had lain in bed, listening to them talk outside on our deck, imagining their faces illuminated only by the frequent lighting of cigarettes—an obvious legacy from their nicotine-addicted Turner forebears. As they laughed frequently and often convulsively, I knew they had uncovered other shared inheritances as well.

Loss has its own particular weight, and after a while I could no longer bear just sitting in the front pew waiting for the service to start. I got up and walked back up the aisle to greet a few friends I had passed on the way in.

A tall, attractive woman probably in her late sixties approached me. She was too old to be a classmate but too young to be a friend of my parents. Her brown hair fell beyond her shoulders, necklaces were draped at varying lengths on her chest, and lightly tinted aviator sunglasses shaded her large eyes. As I quickly scanned her face, she said, "Amy Turner?"

I did a double take. "Patsy Ribner?"

She smiled. "Yes."

There were so many other things I could have said (we hadn't communicated since 1972, my year in Switzerland after high school), but I immediately blurted out, "Isabella James?"

With no hint that she thought my question unusual, she nodded her head in recognition and responded, "Yes."

No one I knew had contacted Patsy Ribner. No one I knew, including Harold, had seen her for over forty years. Was I hallucinating? Had I, months earlier, unearthed her spirit in my archaeological dig for Harold?

But the service was beginning, and there was no time to talk.

———

When Jim asked if anyone else wanted to speak toward the end of the service, I was surprised to see Patsy walking toward the lectern.

She began by saying that when she looked at us, she saw not adults in their fifties but her students, beautiful sixteen-year-olds of whom she was still so fond. We laughed at her stories, many that I had forgotten, including the time a friend and I saved her job by getting our parents to intervene with the principal. And if I had somehow conjured her up, she returned the favor, because after she described Harold at sixteen—how his charm, intellect, arrogance, sensitivity, and preternatural gifts as a writer set him so clearly apart—he, too, sat among us.

Perhaps Patsy had recognized all those years earlier what wouldn't occur to me until I found Harold's poem to our father—that Harold was best appreciated through poetry—because she closed her remarks with an excerpt from a Wordsworth poem:

> What though the radiance which was once so bright
> Be now for ever taken from my sight,
> Though nothing can bring back the hour
> Of splendour in the grass, of glory in the flower;
> We will grieve not, rather find
> Strength in what remains behind;
> In the primal sympathy
> Which having been must ever be;
> In the soothing thoughts that spring
> Out of human suffering;
> In the faith that looks through death,
> In years that bring the philosophic mind.

Although Patsy was standing alive and well before me, the unexpectedness of her appearance reminded me of death. It was as though the gods or nature or the powers that be had dropped her into my life just as suddenly as another person could be—or in the case of Harold and my nephew, Tom, had been—plucked from it. And yet the events all seemed connected, in a way. Ever since my accident, I couldn't escape the feeling that I was in a plotline that someone else was creating. As if the gods were writing my story, taking time that I couldn't imagine they had to include all the details, foreshadowing, and humor that would entice a reader to keep turning the pages. Except I wasn't just the reader. I was also the main character who, with the turn of each page, was being led along to an end I couldn't foresee and still feared. And where would I be then?

From the moment I had crossed that street, having just finished *Change Your Brain, Change Your Life*, and then had my head smashed on the pavement to find myself three hours later in the hospital watching a parade of Buddhist monks, I had wondered whether the accident had been one final attempt to get me to understand the message that had been sent to me a thousand times before in more subtle forms: "Give up—you are not in control!"

There had been so many unfoldings that had followed that day—Harold's death, meeting Isabella, Patsy's reemergence. I recognized that whoever was controlling my life was much better equipped than I, whose only tool, like my mother's, was a white-knuckled grip.

Grace. I doubt I used that word when I next saw Isabella. I would've been afraid that I sounded like some spiritual poseur. But I do think I wondered out loud to her, "But why me and why now? How could I deserve this?"

———

Although I knew I should write a thank-you note to Patsy, I couldn't bring myself to face the emotions it might resurrect. But eight months later, my sense of social obligations won out and I began what I assured myself would be a short message. I didn't want to risk reexperiencing Harold's loss (or subjecting myself to the grammar check of a teacher whose red marks still haunted me from the box in our basement where I had packed away that high school paper on *Alice in Wonderland*). But I soon found myself covering more ground—Harold's death, my accident, the Buddhist monks, and the strange circumstances of meeting Isabella, among other topics.

As I reread my note in a final attempt to catch any stray run-ons or other grammatical errors that might have eluded me, I discovered the other gift that Harold's memorial had given me: I had finally done what my therapist, Barbara, and Isabella—and, thirty-five years before them, my father—had urged me to do. I had started to "get it down."

15

MY FATHER'S RENAISSANCE

BY 1982, MY MOTHER NO LONGER WANTED THE PHYSICAL and financial burdens of maintaining a house as large as 35 Valley. By that point, we children had moved out, each of us supporting ourselves to varying degrees. Louise was living in New York City and pursuing an acting career; Harold may have been either "boarding" at Sarah Lawrence or living in an apartment in Bronxville with Jimmy, who was teaching at a private boys' school in the city; and I was married to Ed and practicing law in Riverhead. And so my parents sold the house and moved into a two-bedroom apartment in a complex in Bronxville about five minutes away from 35 Valley.

I wasn't optimistic about their move. With an area of about 6,000 square feet, 35 Valley had been just large enough to accommodate the writing habits of my father and the distance from each other my parents required. But the presence of even one houseguest could destroy that delicate homeostasis. My father, kind and generous in so many respects, had been forced to accept the habits of his family, but had absolutely no tolerance for even the most inoffensive quirks of others who might be in the house. He once pleaded with my mother to ask the daughter of a family friend who was spending her senior year living with my parents to leave because he could not bear the misspellings in the phone messages she left for him. My mother's solution, eminently practical, was simply to tell the girl not to answer the phone.

But the personal habits of Reza, a Bangladeshi man in his twenties who came to 35 Valley at my father's invitation, posed a much greater threat to my father's equanimity. The last straw for my father was that every morning Reza dumped practically a cupful of sugar on his cereal, oblivious to his starving countrymen 7,800 miles away. My father considered this such an egregious moral violation that he could no longer live with Reza. But rather than ask Reza to leave or, as my mother suggested, simply avoid the breakfast room when Reza was eating cereal, my father moved into the Yale Club in New York City. When he refused to come home for Thanksgiving if Reza was still there, my mother located the man's distant relatives and paid for his round-trip bus fare so he could enjoy his first Thanksgiving with them in Georgia. By the time Reza returned from that trip, my mother had arranged mutually acceptable plans for Reza to leave and my father to return.

Even if my parents didn't have any houseguests, I knew their marriage could never survive the frequent daily contact of living in an apartment. I gave it a year. But even with my mother spending that winter in Key West, their marriage was over in ten months.

My father moved out—only two miles away, but it may as well have been a thousand. At my first visit, I wondered if his lifelong struggle with depression had now become manifest in the form of his new home: a dark one-bedroom apartment on the ground floor of a three-story house located in the commercial district of a sad-looking blue-collar town.

Worried about how he'd manage on his own, I'd come as soon as I could. By then he'd unpacked his belongings, which appeared to be limited to books (Emerson, Yeats, Frost, Pound, and Silone, among others) that filled two large bookshelves, a few items of clothing that hung in the closet, and one household item, an old Mr. Coffee that sat on a small area of grayish Formica next to the electric stove. I asked him whether he had anything for the kitchen, like a pot or dishes.

"No, Ame—it hadn't occurred to me," he said, a look of self-awareness lighting his face. He was an almost seventy-year-old man who to me in that moment looked as out of place and un-prepared for living in this apartment as a zebra. "I guess I'd better get some."

And so we took the first shopping trip I could remember taking together since I was five when we went to the garden store to buy seeds for the corn we were going to plant in our sub-urban backyard. We bought dishes, flatware, two pots, and a bath mat.

Perhaps because I simply couldn't imagine my father clean-ing his own apartment, I passed the shelves of cleaning supplies without a thought. It wasn't until the landlord paid a visit to tell him that the apartment was too dirty that my father bought some supplies. He later called to tell me that he had cleaned the bathroom and mopped his kitchen floor, just as his landlord had shown him how to do. I could hear the pride in his voice, as though he were talking about a piece of writing that had gone well for him.

I, too, should have been proud of him. He was, at age seventy, finally on his own—free of the dependence that had been, he'd tell me many years later, one of his greatest problems. I had accepted the narrative of success that my mother had used during my childhood and adolescence to describe my father's trajectory from business to earning a PhD, but I still sensed a trace of failure in his inability to contribute meaningfully to our family's support and maintain the emotional stability required for regular employment. When I had been desperate to prop up my view of him at other times, I could, despite choking on my own elitism, look to his admission to Yale and its most exclusive club, as well as at his close friends from college, one of whom was a US Supreme Court justice. But I hated picturing him barely scraping by on his small trust fund in that dingy apartment, scrubbing the bathtub on his hands and knees. I winced at my snobbery.

Yet my father continued to speak cheerfully about his domestic endeavors, to marvel at how our housekeeper, Doretha, had been able to do it all so expertly, and to ask me, with no trace of embarrassment, things like how to interpret a utility bill.

On one of these occasions, I was tempted to answer in the way he had whenever any of us asked him for help with our schoolwork. As a high school senior, I knew that consulting him on an assignment would inevitably result in my feeling humiliated. But one night I was so stymied by an English assignment that was due the next day that I decided to risk it.

"Dad, do you know what the green light means in *The Great Gatsby*?"

"Oh, Ame, what? *The Great Gatsby*? Of course. Wait, you don't know what the green light means? Did you read the book?"

"Yeah, Dad, I have an assignment on it."

"Really, you've read the book, but you don't know?"

"Uh-huh, yeah."

"Are you sure?"

At this point, I would have looked like a little tomato—any exposed skin red with embarrassment and my shoulders hunched forward into a ball of shame. But my father never seemed to notice this, and just as I was on the verge of sneaking away, he would smile and say, "Well, in that case let me see if I can help you."

You knew you were in trouble if he turned to the shelf behind him to heave the Columbia Desk Reference—which, at a foot thick, must have weighed ten pounds—onto the desktop in front of him. He would select the indented lettered tab for the subject at hand and then, if it was anywhere past *D*, use both hands to heave the gray cover and unwanted pages back, revealing a wingspan that covered half of his desk.

After carefully lifting each tissue-paper page until he reached his destination, he would slowly move his index finger down the margin and then stop suddenly, his square-edged fingernail perfectly underlining the sought-after word. He would read what was written and then rephrase it in more complicated terms, so that you were more confused than when you started. But whether due to the comfort I took in the sound of the tissue-paper pages as they softly fluttered down to meet the rest or to the absolute confidence in my father's voice, I kept returning to ask questions.

Early on I knew that to ask him questions in front of others would be a mortifying experience, but after seeing the movie *Zelig*, I wondered if I'd missed the opportunity to instantaneously transform myself into "the brain" I'd always wanted to be. When a group of Melville scholars ask Zelig about *Moby Dick*, he is so terrified of having to admit he hasn't read the "greatest American novel" that he suddenly metamorphoses into a brilliant in-

tellectual and astounds his lunch companions with original insights into the book. (Soon he's capable of resembling anyone he
stands next to, from obese men to Chinese fortune-tellers.) My
father, who'd earned a master's degree in English literature, considered himself an authority on *Moby Dick*, but I never had the
confidence to discuss it with him. Instead, I avoided the subject
and delayed reading the book until my father had been safely
dead for three years and I was sure he could not return to inter-
rogate me on the subject.

So, when confronted with my father's questions on his Con
Ed bill, I wanted to respond, "What, Dad, you've never read a
utility bill?" But I stopped myself. (I want to think that I did so
out of compassion, but perhaps it was the product of my lifelong
fear of "getting Dad upset.")

I was concerned that he couldn't manage the struggles of
daily living on his own, and I felt sorry for him. But as he
thanked me for clarifying the bill, I realized that he was happy in
his new surroundings and that perhaps there had been an upside
to his dark, Calvinist upbringing. Although his parents had allowed their children no play on Sundays unless it involved the
Bible, no fun on any other day unless accompanied by guilt, and
no displays of affection unless toward pets, they had also allowed
absolutely no self-pity.

And my father hadn't explicitly asked for my help, or for my
sympathy. I had simply shown up. As usual, I'd been worried
about him—a state familiar to me since early childhood.

My father's independent life was relatively short-lived. In
retrospect, it would look as though he'd been thrown like a slow-
motion boomerang, because six months later he was living in
Bronxville with another Virginia in the same apartment complex

where my mother still lived. There were, however, two critical and most promising differences: this apartment had four bedrooms, and this Virginia was not his wife.

The second Virginia (called by my mother, jokingly, "the younger woman," because she believed she was a year younger than her, and by everyone else as "Geanie") could not be described as "new." She and her family had been neighbors and friends for the entire time we lived at 35 Valley, and Geanie had moved to the apartment complex after her husband died. She had invited my parents to dinner on several occasions, but she and my father did not get involved with each other until after he moved out of the complex. When she invited him over after he and my mother separated, my father walked to Geanie's—now a four-mile round trip to and from his apartment. Even if he'd had a car, I'm not sure he would have used it. The story goes that one evening another dinner guest asked my father why he didn't just stay the night instead of making that long walk in the dark—so he did.

Worried that it might not work out, I arranged and paid for the storage of his furniture.

In Geanie's apartment, surrounded by the evidence of her prolific and varied artistic career—oil paintings, watercolors, vibrant geometric needlepoints, playful wooden "creatures"— and barely a three-minute walk from the apartment where his relationship with my mother and any hope of creative expression had so recently been withering, my father began to flourish.

I believe he experienced this renaissance because it was the first time in his life (or at least in a very long time) that he had been both loved and in love at the same time. Geanie's devotion to him seemed to come with only two conditions: that he confine his writing to one large bedroom, and that he remember to turn off the stove after he boiled water for the tea that, alternating with coffee, he drank all day.

Thinking of my mother's experience of living with my father, one day I asked Geanie whether his quirks drove her crazy. She replied, "Absolutely not. He's handsome, thin, has a full head of hair—what's not to love?"

In Geanie's apartment, my father began his mornings sitting at the breakfast room table drinking three or four mugs of black tea, which gradually prepared his body for the flood of caffeine from the pots of black coffee that he drank throughout the rest of the day. As he sipped, he drew rounded, ashen swirls, black to gray—circles, crescents, and cups—on the artist's nine-by-twelve sketch pad in his lap.

What began as mere "doodles" gradually took a more recognizable form.

One morning when I was visiting, he looked up, graphite nub in hand, and said, "Buttocks, Ame, women's buttocks. I don't know why. But that's what I draw."

If that is how a typical day during his renaissance began, it generally ended in their bedroom—Geanie sitting on their bed, needlepointing in riotous color, and my father sitting nearby in a straight-backed chair, newspaper spread at his feet to catch the wood shavings that fell as he whittled. With the same knives he used on his never-ending quest for lead that would yield a *"New Yorker*–worthy" story, he began for the first time to carve something other than pencils: ballet dancers. Soon it was not enough to rely on pictures of Nijinsky as a model, so he began weekly ballet classes in a dance studio above Times Square. If he was self-conscious doing pliés at the barre with aspiring young actresses, he never let on.

Over time his charcoal swirls suggested an artist's touch and his wooden forms a dancer's fluidity. Whether that was due to the praise Geanie lavished on them, the expensive framing she financed, the unquestionable excellence of the work they were displayed alongside on the apartment walls—products of her own efforts—or my father's actual talent, I could never be sure. I was certain, however, that the clouds under which he had labored for most of his life had parted.

———

Soon after he moved in with Geanie, my father began weekly expeditions to Lincoln Hospital in the South Bronx. Why he made these visits is unclear, but I suspect it was his reaction to living in this new environment. On the one hand, his social conscience (or his Calvinist upbringing, or both) would have required that if he were going to live in the relative luxury of Geanie's apartment, he should surround himself with some serious suffering, if only once a week. But it may also have been Geanie's warmth and affection that inspired him to offer the same comfort to others. And so, in his mid-seventies, my father finally learned the value of hugging a child.

Each week, he would take the train to Harlem's 125th Street station and walk the mile and a half across the Third Avenue Bridge and through the streets of Mott Haven (notorious at that time for its crime and poverty) to 149th Street in the South Bronx. It was futile to suggest he wear a warm coat, as he rarely wore anything heavier than a tweed sports jacket and a long wool scarf.

At first I was confident that Geanie and I could convince

him to take a cab rather than walk through those neighbor-
hoods, but no matter how hard we pleaded or how many times
we offered to pay the fare, he refused. Thinking it would calm
our fears, he told us that one morning a young Black man
blocked his path, shouting, "Hey, man, what you doing up
here?" When my father answered that he was a volunteer at
Lincoln Hospital, the young man said, "Yeah? Okay, man, but
you better be careful," and then accompanied him for a few
blocks. My father never told me what they talked about, if anything, but apparently my father's instincts were right, because
he never had any difficulties or at least never reported any.

If my father was seeking suffering, he surely found it on
the hospital's tenth floor, where "boarder babies," born to
crack-addicted mothers, experienced the hell of withdrawal as
they awaited foster care placement that rarely came. Along
with the other volunteers, mostly elderly women of color, my
father would sit in the neonatal ward for hours, holding babies.

One night he called to tell me about it.

"Ame, it's just amazing. The nurses showed me how to do
it. If you hold the babies close to your body and rock gently,
they stop crying. So I just sit there hugging them."

"That's great, Dad," I said. "That's so nice of you."

"You know," he said, lowering his voice to a confessional
tone, "I just didn't know that hugging babies was so
important."

"Wait—really? You didn't know hugging babies was important?" I was tempted once again to do what he would have
done when I was growing up: repeat the question a few more
times, sigh, reach for the old Columbia Desk Reference, me-
thodically leaf through its pages, and then read aloud—with

great authority and condescension—an entry entitled "The Essentials of Parenting." But, of course, I did no such thing.

"Well, Ame," he said softly, regret tingeing his voice, "I just wish I'd known that when you-all were little. I would have hugged you little guys. It's just that back then we were told not to hug babies—that it wasn't good for you."

Could that possibly be true? And had I never been hugged as an infant? I'd spent decades in therapy unearthing the emotional impacts of my childhood. But without the benefit of this disturbing revelation, I wondered if I understood myself at all.

I reached for the kitchen counter, as if to steady myself. Tears brimmed, my eyelids burned, but I didn't want to cry; I knew my father felt bad enough. To distract myself, I tried to imagine Matthew and Peter, then building a LEGO tower on the kitchen table, with a parent like my father. I thought it would be a far less disturbing prospect since they were hugged all the time. But I was wrong. Even in the hypothetical, it was too pathetic to conjure. There wasn't a stack of Columbia Desk References in the world that would make me feel better, and I ended the conversation as quickly as I could.

"Well, Dad, it's great you're doing that now."

Although I had no reason to doubt that my father had finally learned the value of hugging children, proof nevertheless arrived in the Retired and Senior Volunteer Program's annual calendar that year. There he appeared in an eight-and-a-half-by-eleven-inch photograph, the seventy-seven-year-old pinup for January, wearing a paper hospital gown over his tweed jacket, sitting in a large wooden chair next to his fellow volunteer, Monserrat Bones, smiling down at the tiny infant cradled in his arms.

———

The emotional comfort of living with Geanie may also have helped my father to find the courage to engage in his riskiest act of protest—and by doing so experience what he believed was the divine.

After supporting the Black hospital workers' strike at Lawrence Hospital in 1965, my father continued his political activism, engaging in civil rights protests and anti-war demonstrations. Although my mother shared his political views, her active participation stopped after the hospital strike. She would do what she could through helping individuals and donating to causes. So I stepped in to support him, once again.

As a high school junior in 1970, I was excited to accompany him to the National Moratorium protest in Washington, DC. We traveled on the bus sponsored by the Columbia University Department of Library Science, where my father was a graduate student.

After standing around in a crowd for a few hours, my father suddenly sat down on the grass, exhaled, and, with one side of his mouth hitched up in an embarrassed half smile, said, "I guess the heat's getting to me, Ame . . ."

Since he never complained about physical discomfort, I was worried, but I was also grateful to have this opportunity to assume a caregiving role. We had no water with us, so, buoyed by the importance of my mission, I mustered the courage to ask a woman in a nearby group if I could have a cup of the water she was dispensing from a red-and-white cooler.

I sprinkled a few drops of water on a scarf I retrieved from my faded yellow knapsack and handed the cup to my father.

"This will make you feel better too, Dad," I said as I wrapped the folded scarf around his forehead and tied the ends at the back of his head. There's a favorite photo I have of the two of us—my father wearing his headband, me wearing my red-and-white-striped bell-bottoms and an oversize men's shirt, and another graduate student, in jeans and a T-shirt, holding a fifteen-foot-long black banner with white letters that read, "Librarians against the War."

By the eighties my father had become interested in nuclear disarmament. Never deterred by the disapproval of other people, he had submitted a notice to the *Yale Alumni Magazine*'s class notes for 1937, inviting his "classmates to join [him] in a non-violent, civil disobedience action against our nuclear arms establishment. One likely sight [sic] is the Riverside Research Institute, a nuclear think tank in Manhattan." It appeared between two classmates' notices, one of which announced pride in losing twenty-five pounds and the other reporting on boat racing and "peripheral involvement in right-wing activities."

By the time my father moved in with Geanie, he had joined Kairos, an organization that several peace activists had founded. The most notable among them was Father Daniel Berrigan, the Jesuit priest and poet known for his Vietnam War protests, one of which involved the destruction of draft files that led to his imprisonment (along with the rest of the "Catonsville Nine"). Once a week my father would take the train into New York City and meet in a sparsely furnished apartment on the Lower East Side with others of all ages for an evening of prayer and discussion.

In the beginning, my father's involvement had mainly been in support at various demonstrations or "actions." He also took on for himself a ministry of sorts, writing weekly letters to the

Plowshares members who were serving time for their civil disobedience. His letters to Sister Anne Montgomery and other nuns serving time in federal prisons for protests at nuclear facilities were humorous, literate, and uplifting, and included poetry, pictures of dancers or something else that struck his fancy, and news of the organization. He often sent copies to his children; although I was proud of his efforts, they were also an uncomfortable reminder that as a practicing lawyer and mother of two, I was doing very little to further the chances for world peace. My father never seemed to judge my lack (at that time) of activism, but the personal example he'd set over the previous thirty years was enough to make me feel guilty.

Kairos members never pressured my father to do anything more than serve in a support capacity. You took on your own level of risk as you felt called upon to do so. For years my father would accompany other Kairos members to protests where they did things like throw their own blood on the doors of the Riverside Research Institute.

The demonstrations became routine: the police would be called; the demonstrators would be driven away in a van to a courthouse in lower Manhattan, where they would wait on a bench for most of the day until they were called before a judge; the judge would accept their guilty pleas for trespassing or disorderly conduct; and the court would release them. If a fine was imposed, they would pay it.

When the Riverside Institute moved its offices, Kairos turned its attention to the USS *Intrepid*, the aircraft-carrier-turned-museum that had recently arrived at a pier in New York City. This would be a riskier action, because at a federal facility even symbolic efforts to damage property or interfere with operations promised a tangible form of punishment, not the slap on the wrist the actions at Riverside had elicited.

One day, without mentioning it to anyone, my father joined the group at the *Intrepid*. This time they were handcuffed, arraigned, and ordered to return for trial in two weeks.

I didn't learn about his arrest until my father called to discuss the logistics for his and Geanie's upcoming weekend visit.

"Hi Ame, Geanie and I will be driving out on Friday. I'm not sure what time we'll leave because I'm still waiting to find out if I can bring my medications to Rikers Island."

"What? Where?"

"Rikers Island, honey. I'm probably going there on Monday. They won't let me take my reading glasses, but I think they will allow some medications."

I knew the day might come when we would be forced to have a painful conversation about him moving to a nursing home—but a jail? And not just any jail: the notorious Rikers Island? If I hadn't been so terrified of what would happen to him there, I might have seen the material for the darkest of humor. But I could feel the heat rising to my cheeks and the buzz of anxiety beginning to circulate—the familiar state of worrying.

Monday was his trial date. I pleaded with him to hire an attorney, told him that I would find a lawyer for him immediately, that Ed and I would pay for it. But he wouldn't hear of it.

"No, thanks, honey. Kairos members don't hire attorneys. The point is that we are trying to make a statement—attorneys would defeat the purpose. Anyway, I wouldn't retain an attorney when the rest of them won't have one. I just have to accept it."

His only defense, "justification," was not recognized under federal law. We both knew he'd be convicted. Although I couldn't imagine a seventy-seven-year-old being sent to jail, I took him at his word that more experienced Kairos members were certain they'd be sentenced to a (probably short) prison term. And, as a lawyer, I did know that the courtroom could be full of surprises.

"Dad," I blurted out, "aren't you afraid?"

"Yes, I am, honey, I am."

———

The weekend went as well as could be expected when the subtext was a "send-off to Rikers Island" party. As usual, I tried to avoid my anxiety by finding the humor. What do you serve your father for his last dinner before jail? Are there appropriate gifts for this occasion? Is there a book, perhaps *Rikers Island Rules of Etiquette* or *What to Expect When You're Expecting Imprisonment*? We couldn't talk about the situation much, as Matt and Peter—two and five at the time—always seemed to be within earshot. It would have been far too alarming for them to learn that their grandfather was going to jail, and I wasn't willing to pretend in conversation that Rikers was just another island like nearby Shelter Island.

One night after dinner we stayed at the table on the brick patio late enough for Peter to finally be dozing in my arms, Matt to be listening sleepily, his head resting against Ed's shoulder, and the candles and occasional firefly to be providing the only light. As he had a million times before, Dad got up abruptly.

"Just a moment, I have to get something. I'll be right back."

Would it be *Beowulf*, which he'd long ago read to me and my siblings at a family dinner? A gift?

When he returned to the table, I was relieved to see him carrying his well-worn paperback of poetry, his index finger already marking a place, dividing the thick volume in two. Without his usual introductory interrogation ("Do you know this poem? Really, no? Never read it? It's very important, let's see . . ."), he said, "I just want to read you this. It's by Auden, 'September 1, 1939,' one of my favorites."

I sit in one of the dives
On Fifty-second Street
Uncertain and afraid
As the clever hopes expire
Of a low dishonest decade:
Waves of anger and fear
Circulate over the bright
And darkened lands of the earth,
Obsessing our private lives;
The unmentionable odour of death
Offends the September night . . .

And he finished:

Defenceless under the night
Our world in stupor lies;
Yet, dotted everywhere,
Ironic points of light
Flash out wherever the Just
Exchange their messages:
May I, composed like them
Of Eros and of dust,

Beleaguered by the same
Negation and despair,
Show an affirming flame.

———

When we said goodbye on Sunday afternoon, I begged my father one more time to let me contact a lawyer for him, said it wasn't too late for Ed and me to find a law school friend to appear with him the next morning and ask for an adjournment until we could retain a defense lawyer knowledgeable in the field. With a hint of that "affirming flame," or perhaps a tear, or maybe both, glittering in his eye, he didn't hesitate: "No, thanks anyway, I'll be okay, honey."

I was nervous all day. No call. No word. I pictured him being loaded into the paddy wagon in his orange jumpsuit, out of habit thanking the guards and saying "excuse me" as he sat down on the bench next to the inmates to whom he would be chained. I had to keep apologizing to people in my office. When asked why I was so distracted, my response—"I'm waiting to hear if my father is going to Riker's Island"—got some strange looks.

The call came that night. I was so surprised to hear my father's voice that it took me a moment to speak. "Dad, I can't believe it. Did the trial get adjourned or something?"

"We had the trial, and I don't know how to explain it. The judge asked me if I had anything to say before he sentenced me, and I just got up and began speaking. I know I started with justification, US foreign policy, the horrors of nuclear warfare, Hiroshima, but pretty soon I just felt some presence take over. It felt . . . well, honey, it felt almost like God, something divine. I don't remember what I said. It just came. All I know is that when I finally stopped talking, the judge looked me in the eye and said, 'Mr. Turner, I cannot argue with what you have said.' Then he banged his gavel and said, 'Not guilty.' Ame, I was so stunned I just stood there until he said, 'You can leave now, Mr. Turner.'"

My hunched shoulders relaxed as my worry dissolved into relief—for both of us—that he wouldn't go to jail. And I was happy, too, that he had successfully defended himself in a case that probably no lawyer could have won for him. For a moment I thought of that Thanksgiving vacation when he'd told me he hadn't been able to get through law school. But I could tell from the softness and wonder in his voice that for him the most important part of the experience had been the sense of divine assistance.

16

SOMATIC EXPERIENCING

IN 2012, TWO YEARS AFTER THE ACCIDENT, I WAS STILL seeing Isabella every week. She had begun training in Somatic Experiencing (SE), a psychobiological method for resolving the aftermath of trauma. The theory is based in part on how mammals release the effects of a threatening experience: When facing danger, they instinctively mobilize huge amounts of energy to fight, flee, or freeze. Once the threat is gone, they discharge the energy through involuntary movements such as shaking, trembling, or breathing deeply. Once the animal shakes off that energy, its nervous system returns to balance.

People, on the other hand, have the capacity to reason and repress and often (consciously or unconsciously) ignore their innate capacity to reset the nervous system. As a result, undischarged stress is stored in the nervous system, where it can lead to a wide array of health problems.

To help a person release the unprocessed energy, SE practitioners like Isabella use, among other tools, "pendulation" and "titration," the process of guiding a person back and forth between areas of comfort and discomfort in the body. By momentarily tapping into and then out of physical sensations they've been avoiding, clients are supposed to experience more openness and flow and their trauma eventually becomes "unstuck." If the practitioner allows the client to linger too long in an area of discomfort, she runs the risk of reactivating the client's nervous system, or in other words, compelling it to reexperience the trauma. Thus, the practitioner must be sensitive enough to recognize the early signs that a system is approaching its limit for discomfort—subtle shifts in body language or physiology, which will differ for each person due to the unique features of their nervous systems and underlying traumas.

The SE treatments were simple and foreign to me. Unlike psychotherapy, which focuses on talk, so familiar to me it could feel like routine conversation, SE focuses almost exclusively on the physical. Initially, I could barely detect any internal bodily sensations, other than the unmistakable stomach growl, and when I could, I felt silly doing so. Over years of therapy, I'd been trained to look for psychological insight—the "right" or most plausible interpretation for my feelings. But whenever (and it was often) I veered off into self-analysis, Isabella would redirect my attention: "It's not about the story, Amy. Tell me what's happening in your body."

As I would understand later, this process cultivates a "felt sense"—an internal awareness that promotes "embodiment"—a feeling of being at home in one's body. I had been somewhat skeptical at first, yet undoubtedly I felt lighter, less burdened after each session, as though some dense area of clutter within me had been removed, leaving more space and oxygen.

In one session, Isabella asked me to move my head to the left very gradually—in "micro movements," as she referred to them. It was no surprise that as a result of my accident, the range of motion in my left shoulder and neck was much more restricted than it was on my right side. But moving in slow motion, I noticed sensations—a subtle vibration in my abdomen, a quickening pulse, a sizzling through my limbs—that were vaguely familiar.

As Isabella guided me back and forth between the areas of comfort and pain, I realized that the resistance I was experiencing was not just physical. I did not want to move to the left. It felt dangerous somehow.

A moment later, I was lying once again on that pavement—buzzing, probably from shock, and desperate to shut out what was happening on my left side, where crouching EMTs huddled and discussed my injuries in serious-sounding medical terms: cognitive function, trauma, spinal injury. *What if I'm brain dead?* I wondered. I did not want to hear their muffled voices discussing my symptoms or prognosis, did not want them touching me, prodding me, uncovering some horrible injury. But on the right side was the woman with the soothing Irish lilt reassuring me that I would be fine. She felt safe.

Isabella asked me to stretch my arms straight out in a 180-degree angle. My right arm moved easily, but my left arm resisted. It didn't hurt, but it felt wrong somehow. She told me to move my left arm in any way I was comfortable. I lifted it straight up, a few inches from my neck. My right arm was still outstretched, as she'd asked. Although I was self-conscious in this position, I felt exhilarated. When I looked up at the space between my outstretched arms, I recognized it as the field of vision I'd had as soon as the truck was pulled off me—the elms to my right growing taller against a 90-degree slice of blue sky. That is where I had wanted to be. That is where I had felt safe.

The pain in my left shoulder began to subside.

"Isabella, that was such an amazing feeling as I looked up

between my arms . . ." I still felt a trace of exhilaration as I folded my hands in my lap.

"Where did the truck hit you again, exactly?"

"Kind of just below my left shoulder."

"See if you can point to the area, Amy."

I moved my hand in a large circle against my chest, gradually narrowing the arc to an area that seemed to still remember the impact.

"You know, that's your heart."

I shook my head slowly and smiled.

———

I often asked Isabella questions about the theory of Somatic Experiencing. I'd already had enough experience with it to be fascinated, and she was patient with her explanations.

"You know, in SE, there's a view that people keep repeating traumas to give their nervous systems the opportunity to finally release the energy undischarged from the original incident."

"God . . . the truck. Did I help create that?"

"Oh, I am not saying that. Just that this is an opportunity to restore balance to your nervous system."

"You know, I forgot to tell you, but a couple of weeks ago I was crossing the street at the same place in the same crosswalk. I was even carrying dry cleaning. I was about halfway across when I heard someone frantically shouting my name. I swear my heart stopped. I whipped my head around, but no one was there."

"That must have been so upsetting . . . Look what you're doing with your legs."

I was twisting myself into a pretzel again. I uncurled my legs and tried to tell the rest of the story without tensing.

"I just put my hands over my head and crouched down in the middle of the crosswalk. Pretty stupid, now that I think about it . . . but in a few seconds I realized there was no danger and stood up. When I got my bearings, I saw a friend of mine. She'd just been waving at me from the entrance of the café across the street, trying to get my attention to see if I had time for coffee."

"After that experience, it was a good idea to sit for a while," Isabella said.

"Yeah, it was, but the whole time I was thinking about how weird it had been. For those few seconds in the crosswalk, the past two years since the accident had just vaporized. Like I was outside time's boundaries, no past or present. I guess the nervous system has its own kind of timeline."

———

During one treatment, I asked Isabella how she maintained her own emotional balance when she was constantly dealing with her patients' trauma.

"Spaciousness," she replied. "A space inside that is expansive enough for me to hold other people's problems and treat them from a safe distance."

Eventually, I began to understand what she meant. Lying on the table with Isabella's hand gently placed under my lower back (another Somatic Experiencing technique), I often had a sense that my chest was widening, or expanding outward as if being gently inflated. Other times, the energy circulating inside me permeated the boundaries of my body so that I felt as though I were blending into the scented air around me.

Although at that time I didn't feel any spaciousness when I wasn't on the treatment table, I would later wonder if the subtle opening those treatments created was what had allowed for a thought I'd never had before to float to the surface around that time: *Find the newspaper stories of your father's attempted suicide.* The idea came to me as routinely as one more item for the grocery shopping list might—no fanfare, no warning.

"The Ledge" had been accepted family lore for as long as it had been whispered about in our house. I had repeated the story countless times, always mentioning that pictures of my father had supposedly appeared in the press with front-page headlines. But even though I'd only heard my mother's account once in detail, I had never before thought to check the record. It occurred to me now that I could have misheard her and unwittingly conjured up ways to fill gaps in the story over so many years. In truth, what I remembered had a cloudy quality, as if blurred by the anxiety I'd felt while listening to her.

Even my law school training, which stressed above all else the importance of proof, hadn't triggered in me an impulse to search for evidence. Those three years often felt to me like a "mind wipe" designed to erase any feelings or sensitivities that might muddle one's perception of the facts—a kind of scorched-earth policy against the brain. That education had affected more than my approach to the law; years had passed before I'd revegetated the part of my brain where creative instincts and playful irrationality had once sprouted.

Having chosen a profession dedicated to finding and corroborating facts, why hadn't I thought to confirm the details of the family story of my father's attempted suicide? Perhaps I worried that if I'd misunderstood the story, that would mean my father hadn't actually gotten as far as the ledge, or that if he had, a priest hadn't really talked him off, or that the scene hadn't actually been dramatic enough to attract the press—and if that were true, I'd have no excuse for the anxiety that still plagued me. In my perverse calculation, the more harrowing his experience, the easier it was for me to rationalize its emotional impacts on me. With the story tucked away in my imagination, safely shielded from the facts, I could shape the events for whatever emotional purpose they served.

At first, I kept the family secret, too embarrassed to share it with any of my friends. In the small and tight-knit village of Bronxville, my father's attempt and hospitalization had surely been a topic of conversation, and it seemed likely that some of my friends had heard about it.

By the time I entered college, I'd opened up about the event, but the main purpose for talking about it was to give myself some kind of mystique. As a blonde, blue-eyed girl from an affluent suburb, my primary concern was being dismissed as a cheerleader type when nonconformity was the height of cool. I was terrified of being just another suburban Suzy Creamcheese with average intelligence and boring problems. Which was where my father's story became useful, adding an air of the unexpected to my background.

Later, in law school, I rarely mentioned the incident. I'd like to think that I'd matured enough to stop glorifying a painful episode, but it's more likely that I'd simply found a better label—future attorney—to define me.

When I got older, the story became a badge of courage—not

for my father but for me. Despite the psychological impact of my father's attempted suicide and ensuing depression, as a lawyer, mother, and wife, I had faced it all and emerged a pillar of emotional stability. Maintaining that fiction was important to my self-image. After all, I had spent years in therapy talking about my childhood, and I was certain I'd picked over every last bit of debris left by that minefield.

But somehow, despite all that openness, I'd avoided confronting my father's actual experience. Seeing an image of him on that ledge, stepping into his experience as he looked down at the sidewalk, finding out what the priest might have said to him, or perhaps learning that it hadn't happened that way at all, was in all likelihood too disturbing for me to contemplate, too liable to crack that carefully constructed pillar.

Now, however—after my accident, Harold's death, and my treatments with Isabella—I began to feel an urgency to know the facts. Perhaps the accident had provided me with my own self-defining story, and that was allowing me to cling less desperately to my father's. Or maybe since I, too, had faced the prospect of imminent death, it was just a little less frightening to contemplate what my father must have experienced as he looked down from that ledge. Or maybe the impulse was simply a product of the SE treatments, generated by the release of some undischarged stress.

But I started my search in such a state of anxiety that my first two attempts to research the story at the New York Public (as my family always called that library) were a total waste of time. After spending almost three hours on each visit wrestling with every scratched and crackly microfilmed page of every NYC newspaper for the month of December 1957, I found nothing. Just the important stories of the time—failed satellite launch, AFL-CIO infighting, NATO meeting in France.

Of course, it dawned on me, why would an otherwise unremarkable man's attempted suicide on a New Haven hotel ledge beat out these important stories for front-page coverage? After all, there had never been a slow news day in New York City.

I felt foolish telling Ed that I couldn't find the article, especially after two tries. Would even he see me differently if the story hadn't been published? I was starting to worry no press account existed, that my family had made the tacit decision that as long as the event was an undeniable part of our family history, we might as well make it as dramatic as possible, even if it meant exaggerating here and there. Or worse, that we elevated the event to mythical status—front-page news!—in order to justify the lifelong sorrow, depression, and anxiety my father's attempt had spawned.

17

GOODBYE TO TENNIS
AND ALL THAT

SEVENTEEN YEARS AFTER MY MOTHER WARNED ME I'D regret giving up tennis, I had to admit to myself that she might have been right. In 1986, my feelings on joining a country club hadn't changed, but my circumstances had. By then, Ed and I lived next door to her summer home, in the house we'd built on the land she'd given us. Nine months of the year were wonderful, but the three summer months when my mother and I were neighbors were as tough on me and my marriage as anything has ever been. I tried to maintain a balance between what I felt were my obligations to my mother—whose generosity had enabled us to live a mile from the ocean in an area that we could never have afforded otherwise and whose attachment to my children was genuine—and my husband, who accused me of being more concerned about her than him. I told her I would join the Georgica Association and play tennis with her there but reassured Ed that he would be excused from having to act out any of her country club fantasies, like attending the association's cocktail parties and taking up men's doubles. And yes, I now wished I had a decent tennis game.

She was amazingly patient at the beginning. I was sure she

would enjoy some schadenfreude at my missed overheads or my clumsy footwork, or be angry that I was losing games for us, but for the most part she was encouraging. We played as partners in friendly weekend ladies' doubles, but eventually we found ourselves across the net from each other in the finals of the ladies' doubles tournament. She was nothing if not competitive. (After pitching a losing high school game, she had kicked a school door so hard that its glass shattered.) But my partner was equally so, and the trepidations I felt about beating my mother were irrelevant in the face of my partner's determination. After we won, my mother forced a tense smile as we shook hands over the net.

The next year, we found ourselves in the same situation. We had split sets, and my partner and I were up by a game in the third. All I could think about was how angry she would be to lose two years in a row. After last summer's defeat, she'd been insufferable, stomping around her house, muttering expletives periodically through tight lips, and answering questions with only the fewest words possible. Should I really put her through that misery? For what? I didn't care that much, but wasn't tennis supposed to be just a game where each side, related or not, plays their best and the chips fall where they may? Was my mother struggling with conflicted feelings as well? Shouldn't it be more difficult for a parent to maintain the motivation to defeat a child than a child to defeat a parent?

From her glare and clenched teeth, it appeared that her only struggle was with returning the ball. My mind kept racing and my game fell apart. I think my partner knew why I couldn't hit the ball over the net and did not bother to raise her game to compensate for my meltdown. We lost the third set, and when we all shook hands, my mother and I were both relieved, albeit for very different reasons.

A couple of weeks later at a cocktail party, I overheard someone ask her, "Wasn't it difficult to play against your daughter in the finals?" I stopped in my tracks so that I could hear her answer. Would she describe how she battled with competing emotions as I had? I waited.

She paused, as if considering such a question for the first time, and then replied, "No, not really. If I just remember that she's left-handed, I'm alright."

I couldn't contain myself. I swung around, smiling broadly but incredulously. "Mom, are you kidding? I was out there dying, worrying about how you'd feel if you lost again. I couldn't bear it."

She just smiled and repeated that no, it hadn't bothered her. I got some sympathetic looks from the others, but I didn't need them. She couldn't help it: tennis was that important to her, and that was that.

My mother played tennis for the last time in June of 1999, shortly before her seventy-seventh birthday. She was more easily winded and took a longer time changing sides. On the morning after her birthday dinner on June 23, standing across from me at "command central"—her post at the kitchen counter from where she could see all movement in the combined dining and living room areas and, beyond that, the deck outside—she pursed her lips, nodded her head as if to signal the finality of what she was about to say, and with no other introduction, announced, "I have lung cancer."

"My God, Mom, when did you find out?"

"Three weeks ago, about."

"What? How could you have kept it a secret? We've played tennis together. We had so many laughs last night at dinner. I can't believe it . . ." When I heard the cat scratching the screen door, I was grateful for the momentary distraction of having to let her inside. I had no idea what to say next, and the buzzing in my head was making it impossible to think. If I blurted out the fear and sorrow and shock roiling around in my brain, or even attempted to console her, she might end the conversation. She loathed emotional displays and responded to words of comfort the way many others react to an intrusive question: she clammed up and moved on.

As I returned to my stool at the kitchen counter, she broke the silence.

"I didn't want to tell anyone before my birthday. I just wanted to have a happy birthday with my grandchildren. And I haven't really been able to believe it. There was a spot on the X-ray, but I never thought it would be cancer."

"Really?" I asked tentatively. "Mom, you smoked two packs a day for fifty years . . . You didn't think you might get cancer?"

"No, I never did."

We both glanced at the pack of Merits on the counter.

"I'm so, so sorry, Mom." She nodded at me and then quickly reached for her coffee mug. That was the extent of the compassion she was willing to receive and I was willing to risk. I returned to the practical, her preferred domain, and asked whether she'd told my brothers, both of whom were in Iowa, or my sister, who lived in Texas.

"No, you were first since you live here. I'll tell them now."

She turned to leave the room but then reached back toward the counter to pick up her cigarettes, which she slid into the front pocket of her white tennis shorts.

"Do you want me to stay, Mom?"

"Nope," she said. "I guess I'll see you at three when I pick up Matt for his tennis lesson."

———

At first she was adamant that she would see her doctors alone. But fortunately a friend who had survived cancer convinced her that taking someone with her was not a sign of weakness but a necessity, as she'd inevitably be confronted with a barrage of complicated medical options. She finally allowed and later encouraged me to accompany her on her many trips to Sloan Kettering in New York City.

I was grateful my mother had the means to hire a driver because the round trip was exhausting, taking six hours on a good day, and I had to be available on a moment's notice to adjust her oxygen tank in the car. She was not an easy patient at first, and, petulant as a toddler resisting naptime, she struggled against the constantly invading army of nurses and technicians, a losing battle, until she enlisted the support of her surgeon. Her chart notes were telling: "Do not interrupt the patient when she is meditating."

Living nearby, I was able to spend every free moment with her when I was not commuting ninety minutes to graduate school two evenings a week, student teaching every day, and attending (just barely) to the needs of my husband and sons. To my friends, I appeared to be a devoted daughter, but any sacrifices I made were motivated by my own needs as much as by my love for my mother. I was desperate for the peace of mind that would come from knowing I had done everything I could to get closer to her. I couldn't bear the thought of compounding my grief with feelings of regret and guilt.

Although I had Ed's support, stealing that time away from my children, ages ten and thirteen, would trouble me for years.

———

As chemotherapy took its toll and prospects for lung surgery dimmed, my mother had difficulty maintaining her white-knuckled grip. She surrendered to my pleading and ate the meals I or others prepared for her. She relied on me to fix her oxygen tank as she gasped for air. She let me see her pout and cry and moan in pain. She let me help her dress and use the toilet. Her sagging skin, weighed down by fluid rather than the extra weight we'd hoped for, melted underneath my touch. Those clenched muscles, as fundamental to her frame as her skeleton, had finally let go.

Despite her diagnosis, my mother still could not quit smoking. I was surprised when she followed her surgeon's advice to talk to a counselor at Sloan Kettering.

She'd always insisted that for her, action, not conversation, was the way to solve her problems (if she ever had any), so I was surprised and touched that she talked about her session with me.

"You know, I spoke to the counselor today. I was amazed. She said that smoking creates anxiety. I always thought it reduced it."

"Me too," I said. "I think everyone reaches for a cigarette to calm down. I certainly did."

"She asked me to list all the situations where I needed to

smoke. I realized that I always have to light a cigarette before answering the door."

"Really? Even here in Wainscott? The only people who come here are your friends and delivery people."

"I know." She smiled at me as her face reddened. "It still makes me anxious. I always need a cigarette."

Although I managed to keep my jaw closed, my insides dropped. She had been as frightened as the rest of us. Despite all my years of therapy and self-reflection, I had *never* before this moment recognized her anxiety. I hadn't seen it, I reassured myself, because she had hid it *so* well. I looked away to hide the flush of my cheeks. I suppose I'd needed to believe that through her preternatural strength she had conquered fear and every other emotion she considered a sign of weakness. I believed that such strength could, if ever necessary, save me.

My mother's early childhood losses must have been devastating. But now, seventy-three years later, she exhibited for the first time, it seemed to me, the most authentic form of strength: the power to admit her own vulnerability.

She was proud of herself when she quit smoking a week later.

———

On one Friday afternoon in the fall, several months after her diagnosis, I found my mother sitting up in bed, as usual. I had stopped by the teachers' TGIF get-together after school and hoped she wouldn't smell the alcohol on my breath. I would have been embarrassed to admit to a person in the program, especially one who was confronting a fatal disease, that I was the one who needed a drink.

I lay down on her bed and, after a few minutes of chatting, dozed off. When I awoke, she was leaning back against her pillows, her eyes closed, the ends of her mouth suggesting a smile. I nestled deeper into the comforter, yet the warmth that enveloped me seemed to originate elsewhere. Blurred by my half sleep, the edges of time and memory were still soft, and I felt, for a few blessed moments, only the depth of our connection.

———

A week before Christmas, my mother was admitted to Sloan Kettering because her lungs were constantly filling up with fluid. I was fortunate enough to be able to stay nearby in a friend's apartment whenever I needed to. We had hoped that she would be home for Christmas, but the doctors would not allow her to leave. Although she must have known that this would be her last Christmas, she insisted that I spend the day with my family. I took the last bus home and arrived at 2:00 a.m. on Christmas Eve. As I stepped into the darkness and quiet of the deserted street, the lightly falling snow seemed to demarcate a parallel universe safely insulated from the intercom dings, hurried footsteps, buzzing monitors, hushed whispers, and distant groans of the hospital—where people ride elevators that stop at floors that are referred to not by their numbers but by the particular organ treated there, and death's beckoning chatter is a constant.

During the week between Christmas and New Year's, I spent several days at home with my family, confident that my mother was being well cared for: Jim, who had come from Iowa, was visiting her daily, and Harold and Louise and her family would be arriving during that period as well. Still, I made a few day trips to visit her by myself, and on New Year's Eve, Ed, Matt, and Peter joined me.

I was happy that she had lived to see the new millennium arrive: it was the kind of achievement she might want to brag about in heaven. We stopped to buy flowers on the way to the hospital, and as I headed up to the register with a bouquet I'd chosen quickly, Matthew said, "Don't you think we should give her something special?"

I stopped. Matt, the one who watched and listened and said very little, had recognized what the rest of us, in our haste and worry, didn't want to think about: this gift was part of saying goodbye.

"Of course, Matt," I said. "You're right. Why don't you choose the flowers?"

He took his time and finally settled on an orchid, its white blossoms, tinged with light green, bowing gracefully, if mournfully, at the end of two tall, arcing stems.

At the hospital, the four of us walked into my mother's hospital room. Her face brightened at the sight of the orchid, but her eyes misted over when we told her that Matt had insisted on this plant. She understood its significance to him.

———

A few days after New Year's, I returned to the city. Jim, who was staying with my father and Geanie in Bronxville, thirty minutes away by train, was at the hospital too. At times, we spelled each other; at others, we sat in her room together. Until then, the doctors had been confident that my mother could spend her last weeks at home, where all she wanted to do, she said, was to lie on her bed and listen to the children playing in her backyard. But she'd worsened in recent days, and it was now questionable whether she could survive the three-hour ambulance trip to her home in Wainscott.

Jim and I agonized over the decision. As much as we wanted to bring her home, we cringed at the idea of her dying en route, and as much as we were trying to find a bit of comic relief wherever we could, we couldn't run the risk of turning her death into farce—"Oh, no she didn't suffer, really, the traffic on the LIE wasn't that bad," or "I think she was comfortable when she died. She did always like Exit 53."

On January 7, the doctors said she had just a day or two left. The surgeon sat with me as I made the calls to my other siblings. That afternoon, sitting at the end of her bed, I said, "Mom, I'm going to miss you."

Her eyes closed, she replied, "I'm going to miss you too."

———

By the next day, her eyes still closed and breathing slowly, she was not communicating at all. The doctors swore it was her last day, but that day passed, and then another, and with each day, they were more surprised. I stroked her forehead and told her how good she looked.

"Really, Mom, your skin looks great."

The edges of her mouth curved just a little and she whispered, "Thank you."

The next day, she started to mumble under her breath, "Nice shot. Good going." Then, after a disappointed sigh, "Nice try." Her head moved ever so slightly to the left and then the right.

With amused disbelief, Jim and I realized she was watching her last tennis match.

Her doctors were stunned that she kept holding on. And so were we, until Louise figured it out. She and our mother had a strong memory for dates. Louise was the one who realized she must be waiting for January 14, the first anniversary of her brother Tom's death.

When Friday the fourteenth rolled around four days later, we readied ourselves: Jim, at the foot of her bed, softly reading aloud from the Bhagavad Gita, and me at her head, my right hand resting near her heart so that I could feel her pulse as it slowed—beat, pause, beat, pause, no beat, no beat.

I waited one more moment, hoping the silence meant just the beginning of a different rhythm. She had spent most of her life with her jaw clenched, on high alert to defeat a steady stream of opponents—alcohol, suicide, better tennis players. Wouldn't she also struggle with death?

But she didn't need to. As if in deference to the strength my mother had exhibited throughout her life, the end had waited for the day she had chosen. Her seventy-seven years seemed to simply dissolve, as though she'd floated through life and now, seamlessly, into the beyond.

18

PANIC AT THE
NEW YORK PUBLIC

SIX MONTHS AFTER MY FRUITLESS VISIT TO THE NEW YORK
Public, as I was scanning photographs and letters I'd found in my
mother's house after her death, I came across a file I had labeled,
"Dad at the hospital." Amidst the sympathy cards was a sheet of
stationery—"Dominican Fathers, St. Mary's Priory" engraved at
the top—a letter written in perfect Catholic school cursive that
began, "Dear Mrs. Turner, I am Father Keating, the priest who
was involved in what still must be an awful nightmare for you,
Mr. Turner's unfortunate experience last week."

As my hands trembled, an image emerged from the fog that
still obscured the months immediately following my mother's
death in 2000, almost twelve years earlier. I had been sitting
alone on my mother's bed on a freezing gray February day about
a month after she died when I'd stumbled on Father Keating's
letter. My hands had trembled then, too, as I tried to imagine
what it must have been like for her to read the letter for the first
time, her husband catatonic in a mental hospital and her children no doubt screaming around the house. Had she ever reread
it? Or had the letter been tucked away and not opened again
until I had found it after her death?

As I held the letter that February day, feelings of grief and
love seemed to transcend time and distance. I felt that the three

of us—my mother, Father Keating, and me—were reunited, if only for an instant.

I don't know why I hadn't remembered that letter when I was researching at the library. Perhaps it was because I associated it with my mother rather than my father. Now, sitting on my bed, I cried as I marveled how these beautifully written words still had the power to comfort fifty-five years later.

> May I convey my sincere sympathy to you and your four children. I can imagine how hard these days have been for all of you in view of the New York press. It is my hope and prayer that with God's grace you will not allow your minds to exaggerate the ill effects. Please remember we are all called upon to share trying experiences in life, even humiliating ones. It seems that life is like that. Please do not feel that you are marked in any way by what has happened. No, you have too much company among mankind today.

> To turn to a happier note, I am pleased to be able to forward you the best wishes of two of your friends. . . . Both have expressed concern for your welfare and wish they could help in some way. Their sincerity was impressive. That you and your husband have won such respect and sincere friendship is something you can be proud of.

> God bless you, Mrs. Turner, and your children, and may His grace see all of you through this burden. Rest assured of frequent remembrances in my daily Masses.

> Sincerely,
> James Keating, OP

I was so focused on the text of the letter, I didn't at first notice the date at the top: November 17, 1957. No wonder I hadn't been able to find the articles. I had been searching the wrong month.

———

Falling snow dissolved into the slick of Fifth Avenue but left a delicate, loosely knitted veil on the library's staircase. From their ten-foot-high pedestals, the two marble lions gazed toward the eastern horizon, unfazed by the miles of intervening buildings. A regal welcome for all seekers, even those searching for nothing more than a clean bathroom.

For a moment, I hoped the pair might turn me away.

Just inside the entrance was a long, narrow table on which visitors' bags were lined up for inspection. One of two security guards looked up and, when he saw that I carried only a legal pad, waved me through. I knew exactly where to go, and I thought I would be ready for the research—but as I listened to my boot heels click down the long, empty, marble-floored hall to the periodicals room, my heart quickened and I tightened my arms around the yellow legal pad I was hugging against my chest.

The thick, dark wooden door emblazoned in gold with "Room 100" is the only grand feature of the microform periodicals room. Unlike the rest of the library, it is small and unimpressive, a bland mix of metal, cheap wood, and plastic. On the Formica-topped counter to the right of the door sit cups of dark green golf pencils and trays of scattered slips of white paper, the tools for requesting the more obscure newspapers.

The two women sitting behind the counter didn't look up from their reading material as I walked by. A few steps beyond, a young man leaned against the wall, his head bowed, his thumbs tapping on the cell phone in his hands, the library badge at the end of his royal-blue NYPL lanyard resting in the crease between his shoulder blades. To the left and perpendicular to the counter were rows of long, blond wood tables, the first few unoccupied, the last three crowded with microfilm readers of both the mechanical and human varieties. In the back of the room, rows of army-green metal shelving held the shallow trays of cardboard-boxed rolls of microfilm to which visitors had free access.

Having been here twice before to search for the pictures of my father, I easily located the box stamped "November, 1957, *New York Daily News*." As I tried to slide the roll onto the spool, however, I fumbled, both out of fear and clumsiness.

I gave up quickly and asked the young man with the cell phone to help me. If he wondered why a sixty-year-old woman couldn't cope with equally ancient technology, he didn't let on. It was so easy for him; he threaded the film with one hand and with the other held his cell phone up to read texts, mastering at once the old and the new.

Like baseball cards flicking on bicycle spokes, the images of housewives in high heels touting vacuums, mob bosses being pushed into cop cars, and "Negroes" picketing along storefronts sped by. My heart sped as well, and I whisked beads of sweat off my left temple. Forcing a sharp exhale, I told myself that it was just my father's image I was racing toward, not some unknown horror my body seemed to be anticipating. The reminder didn't work. I began to hope that Father Keating had been wrong about the press coverage, that the images speeding by would never make way for a man on a ledge; I realized that it might be easier for me to spend years dismantling a fraud at the foundation of my identity than a minute facing the actual truth. I hadn't realized how terrifying even the prospect of seeing the images would be until this moment.

Suddenly, a white figure in a black void flashed on the screen, different from any other image that had whizzed by. It reminded me of the iconic photograph of Armstrong's first steps on the moon—except this was 1957, not 1969. The possibility of it being my father registered a second later. I pressed the stop button and tried to turn the dial slowly enough to rewind just a fraction. But my hands jittered too much for such a precise maneuver, and the film jerked back and forth, the reel screeching under the glass.

After finally steadying myself, I stopped the machine on the right image and rotated the blue zoom wheel to enlarge it. Almost too afraid to look, I squinted at the screen just long enough to make out the figure standing on the ledge, the fireman's ladder propped up against it, a face in the window, my father's name in the caption, and a few lines of type.

I closed my eyes and inhaled deeply, hoping to stave off the heaviness bearing down on my chest. I had accomplished what I'd set out to do, which was to simply confirm that the newspaper photos existed. Yet I was disappointed. Now that I had finally found the newspaper, I wanted to know more. Why had my father climbed onto that ledge? What had he felt as he stared at the pavement below? What had Father Keating said to him? And, most important, why had he climbed back into his room? Did he want to see his children again, or did he just lose his nerve? And as he was led to the ambulance, presumably surrounded by reporters straining to get one more picture of him, did he wish he had jumped?

But this short article couldn't do that—probably no article, whatever the length, could. Only my father had those answers, and he'd died almost ten . . .

My mind stopped dead, as if it had suddenly screeched to a halt on an empty black slide. My hands and feet, then limbs and torso, began vibrating so intensely that the air around me started pulsating as well. I had the sense I was evaporating, as though my body had lost its power to contain me. Sirens blared louder as they sped closer, as real as if I were on the street, not in the almost soundproof microform room of the New York Public. I was on the verge of hyperventilating.

I felt my father's presence. I knew in my bones that if I opened my eyes, he would be standing before me—either ready to answer my questions or furious I was unearthing images that (as far as I knew) no one in my family, not even my parents, had ever seen. I'd violated our family's code of secrecy and was terrified he'd rail at me—or, worse, appear crushed. But at that moment, I was even more afraid of what this signified about my mental state. Whether or not I saw him when I opened my eyes, I must be going crazy. Crazy enough to conjure his presence, or to have been convinced I could.

I held my breath, squeezed my eyelids tighter shut, and willed myself back to the present, back to my body.

When I finally opened my eyes—the experience had probably lasted three minutes but felt like thirty—nothing had changed. The room was library quiet; the microfilm readers remained in their obedient rows, ready to frustrate any comer; the two ladies behind the desk were still looking down at the papers they were reading; and the man sitting beside me was not my father but the staff member who was still entranced by his phone.

Having just been certain—for an undeniably real moment—that my father might manifest in front of me, reading the newspaper now seemed slightly less daunting. I asked the young man if he could help me print the pages.

Barely glancing up, he positioned the film to print the front-page headline, whose four-inch bold type covered the entire area above the fold: "MUST SPEND TO ARM, SAYS IKE. *Cites 'Red Danger to Free Men.'*"

"Not that," I said. "Sorry, below the fold—there, those pictures and the story in the middle, and then on page fifteen where the story continues."

He focused the viewer, pressed print, and handed me the copies. I still couldn't bear to look at them. Too uncomfortable to stay silent, I waved the papers at the man and (though I cringe at the memory) blurted out, "Look, that's my father fifty years ago—out on the ledge, about to jump."

He glanced at the picture. "Oh jeez, wow," he said, then tactfully returned his gaze to his phone. Just another day at the New York Public.

———

It took weeks before I could even glance at those pages. Just the thought of it made my heart race and my skin flush. As many times as I had talked about my father standing on the ledge, I had never pictured him "pajama-clad" and "barefoot," as the *Daily News* described. Obviously anyone who steps out on a

ledge to contemplate suicide is distraught, but somehow his being in pajamas made his desperation even more palpable. I didn't
even want to contemplate what that meant. Instead, I resorted to
humor, remembering how strictly he had adhered to traditional
standards of appropriate dress, once even firing a psychiatrist
because he refused to take off his baseball cap during a therapy
session. I'd never imagined he'd wear anything so informal for an
act as public as suicide.

When I finally squinted at the pictures, I realized I had never
really visualized the attempt at all. My only interest had been in
how the event had affected me. Picturing the actual attempt
would have meant facing what my father felt—a notion I now
realized had been too scary and painful for me to confront. Usually people, especially those who've spent years in therapy, have
at least some idea of what they're afraid of, even if for just that
instant when the thought breaks the surface of the conscious
mind before being quickly and once again repressed to the
depths from which it escaped. But I must have been so afraid of
knowing my father's experience on that ledge that I made sure
any curiosity about it could never even start the journey toward
consciousness. Not until I saw the microfilm for the first time
and experienced what must have been a momentary panic attack
did I realize how deeply I had buried my fear.

Had I ever allowed myself to wonder about the event long
enough to formulate a picture of it, I'm sure I also would never
have expected him to have climbed onto the ledge on a sunny
Wednesday morning. Suicides, at least in my imagination, took
place in darkness, or at least on appropriately gloomy days, and
in private. But there was my father, looking down from a fifty-
foot ledge on the fifth floor of the Taft Hotel as "several hundred

Yale students watched from the street below," presumably on their way to their first class of the day. Did my father, who as a Yale student had crossed that campus myriad times twenty-three years before, see himself in them?

According to the newspaper account, "Rev. James D. Keating of St. Mary's [Catholic] Church" was walking by "with two other priests" and "dashed" into the hotel when he saw my father, as the *Daily News* put it, "on his perch"—as if he were getting ready to fly rather than jump. One of the pictures, taken at a distance, showed an indistinct image of Father Keating, a fuzzy black figure with just a hint of white visible at the collar, resting his elbow against the hotel windowsill as he appeared to talk to my father at his left. My father's head was lowered just enough to see the pavement below but not enough to upset his balance, which he appeared to be maintaining by pressing his back, ramrod straight, against the building.

Another picture showed a fireman's ladder extended from the truck and leaning against the building just to the left of the window, at the ready, just in case the rescue needed more than faith in God and the Catholic Church. In the next photograph— "seconds later," according to the account—my father had turned slightly toward Father Keating, pressing his left arm against the building for balance and his right against his face. The caption read, "Turner holds head as if he were deep in thought," but to me it looked as though he was clutching his head in pain. After "twenty tense minutes," the fourth picture showed my father, his back to the camera, raising his left knee onto the windowsill as Father Keating grabbed him by his left shoulder to help him climb back through the window. The caption read, "The crowd applauded."

"Reprieve from Eternity," the headline announced. "Reprieve"—saved from something awful, a punishment; a welcome relief. But is being saved from eternity being saved from a punishment? Couldn't eternity have been a welcomed reprieve from the punishing pain my father must have been experiencing during life?

The *Daily News* had answered my questions about the logistics of my father's suicide attempt and confirmed the family lore of press coverage. I wondered whether another New York City newspaper had covered the story in more detail—but I wouldn't try to find out. If glancing at these few pictures and skimming a short article had put me on the verge of a panic attack, I didn't even want to imagine what a more detailed press account might do to me. I folded the printed copy and put it away, half hoping that I would lose it or that any remaining curiosity would return to the depths where it had, until now, been safely buried.

19

TRAUMA

MY SESSIONS WITH ISABELLA WERE A WEEKLY COMFORT, if not a luxury. By 2013, three years after the accident, I rarely noticed my residual dizziness or shoulder discomfort—as long as I avoided raising my arms above my shoulders, moving my head from side to side, or looking up at a steep angle. I could've discontinued treatment, but I sensed the possibility of a more profound type of mending, though I couldn't explain what that might be.

Lying on the treatment table in that oasis of calm with Isabella sitting beside me, her hand underneath my lower back, I would descend into myself so thoroughly that my body seemed on the verge of melting over the table's edges. Although Isabella said she used the palm of her hand solely to monitor what was occurring within my body, I wondered if it was the energy transmitted by her touch that deepened my experience.

The process felt so magical it was difficult for me to appreciate its scientific basis. As Isabella explained, my parasympathetic nervous system was triggering the more tranquil functions of my body (commonly referred to as the "rest and digest" activities) and restoring balance to my nervous system. I knew all too well that I was more accustomed to operating under the influence of the sympathetic nervous system, which activates the fight-or-flight response—the physiological consequences of feeling threatened or being on guard. In that situation, the system releases cortisol and other stress hormones—which, if the pattern is repeated often enough, will eventually dysregulate the nervous system. Locked in that cycle (Isabella sometimes referred to it as "the red vortex"), a person loses the capacity to return to a settled state. In simpler terms, Isabella would just say that my body was healing itself.

In one session, after my descent into relaxation, I was surprised when Isabella placed needles on the top of my head—precisely where parents are cautioned not to touch newborns. Although Isabella had a gentle touch and used only the finest-gauge needles on me, my head felt tender, and the pinch at the insertion points didn't dissipate as it usually did. After a few minutes, she began the Somatic Experiencing technique of "titrating," guiding me between areas of comfort and discomfort.

"Where do you feel the most settled?" she asked softly.

The area that came to mind wasn't one of my typical answers and seemed strange, if not a little embarrassing. But in the interest of ensuring the efficacy of the treatments, I always tried to be honest.

"Well . . . I guess it's the inside of my right foot, along the arch."

"Nice. Do you associate a color or a texture with it?"

"This is so weird, but I'm seeing my mother's tanned foot outstretched in front of her . . . on the beach. She loved to sit in the sun."

"Can you stay with that?"

"I don't know why . . . but I see a crescent moon, a cradle

shape . . . pale rose . . . It's soft, like fur . . ." My mind drifted off as I imagined the cradle's plushness against my skin.

"And how are the needles now?"

It took me a moment to refocus on the top of my head.

"Wow, I don't feel anything there."

"Good. I'll give you some time to rest while the needles do their work. Okay, Amy?"

I barely heard the door close as Isabella left the room and entered another part of her house. I lay in the semidarkness, soothed by the fragrance of rose essential oil. The sound of classical guitar music faded into the silence; my thoughts seemed to dissolve just as soon as they surfaced. I could feel, if not hear, the low-pitched hum of electricity-like energy circulating within me.

A few moments later, that buzzing flowed outward as well, as though my skin could no longer contain or protect me. Although my boundaries seemed to be slipping away, I felt safe.

Suddenly, I gasped for air. A stone slab bore down on my chest. I tried to sit up to inhale more deeply, but I couldn't stay propped up on my elbows—the stone was too heavy. My heart pounded against the weight. Although some part of me must have been aware there was no stone, I was terrified, completely powerless. I saw the shaded windshield and the dark blue hood of the truck coming toward me . . . but just as it was about to hit me, the truck abruptly disappeared, as though a slide projector had been clicked.

Initially surprised, I realized the image didn't quite fit—I'd been standing, not lying down, when the truck neared. The pressure on my chest lifted, but I was overwhelmed with sadness, not relief. A sob caught in my throat. It occurred to me that I never cried on the day the truck hit me, or for weeks afterward.

I followed the warmth of my tears as they slid down my cheeks and dampened the pillow underneath my head.

I felt the first inkling of a distant memory—like a vague twinge in my mind—but before I could grab hold of it, my chest began to ache. My shoulders hunched forward to protect me, a reflexive but futile response, and I quickly flattened back down onto the table. As the ache spread into my abdomen and limbs, it may have also dredged the depths, because within seconds I recognized this longing, this yearning to be consoled and rescued. I was back in 1957, the year of my father's attempted suicide—back to being my four-year-old self.

Just then, Isabella reentered. "Are you alright?" She must have sensed something had happened.

"I think I am . . . now, anyway. It was all so soothing, and then, out of the blue, I couldn't breathe, couldn't even move. I was facing the truck again and terrified."

"That must have been unsettling."

"Yes, but it shifted to sadness. It was like my body knew what was going on before I did. I realized it wasn't the truck that was the real trauma; it was my father. I was experiencing what I must have felt when my father suddenly disappeared—so vulnerable, such despair. And then being afraid to upset him all those years."

"When those patterns get locked in the nervous system so young, they become deeply rooted," Isabella said as she guided me off the treatment table to a chair by her desk. After taking a seat opposite me, she reached for the water pitcher and filled the cobalt-blue glass that sat on the desk at my right elbow.

"And then I felt this longing to be rescued," I said, "but I knew nobody was coming. Maybe I also sensed my mother's drinking back then, even though I didn't understand it."

As I looked up at Isabella, I glimpsed the human anatomy chart, whose bold black and red Chinese characters always intrigued me, displayed on the wall behind her. For my entire life I'd belittled the role of my body, valuing it merely as a vehicle for staying healthy and serving my vanity. I'd been convinced that it was through the "I" of my mind—in dialogue with a therapist—that if I just dug deep enough, as my father had always advised, I'd unearth the source of my problems. Yet it was undeniable that just a few minutes earlier the physical techniques of Somatic Experiencing and acupuncture had excavated an experience more profound and immediate than any I'd had in therapy. I shook my head as the flush of humility, even awe, warmed my face.

Isabella lifted a small, green-labeled bottle of lemon from the row of other remedies lining the top of her desk and shook a few drops into my glass. "Here, this would be good for you . . . You know, even without the language to express it, young children perceive what's happening around them."

My next thought was punctuated with a physical sensation, like the bounce an elevator sometimes takes after it first lands on its floor. "God, it could've been an awful chain reaction. If my mother had started drinking again, there would have been no one to take care of me. It must have been less painful for me to believe I could save my father and keep my mother from drinking." I took a sip of water from the glass, which felt heavy. "Better for me to stay on guard for signs that he might jump or she might drink—let that constant circuit of anxiety keep me focused."

"That's a terrible toll on the system, to be in that constant state of fight or flight."

The ache I'd felt on the table echoed in my abdomen. "Yes, but feeling that utter vulnerability and despair, the way I did today, would've been way too scary."

Maybe it still is, I thought.

20

THE ZIPLOC BAGS

BY 1999, AT THE AGE OF FORTY-SIX, I'D BEEN AT
the Riverhead law firm for seven years and had managed to cir-
cumscribe my responsibilities so that (with the help of an antidepressant) the anxiety I felt each day was exhausting rather
than paralyzing. Having resigned myself to dreading work for
the rest of my life, nobody was more surprised than I when a
breakthrough finally came to me later that year.

I'd volunteered to teach a weekly sixth-grade social studies
class at the middle school Matt attended. When I'd seen the
notice calling for volunteers to teach a six-week class in the
newsletter he brought home, I knew it wouldn't be an opportunity to spend more time with him: Matt wasn't in that grade.
And I wasn't particularly interested in the topic, or in spending
forty-five minutes with twenty-five eleven-year-olds. But something about teaching appealed to me. In elementary school, my
favorite after-school game had been to corral the younger
neighborhood kids and make them listen to my lectures on
various topics, such as when to cross a street (which I got
wrong but fortunately didn't lead to any casualties), tricks for
spelling multisyllabic words, and simple arithmetic. And
teaching did run in the family. After his breakdown my father
briefly taught English, though at the college level; my mother

had a knack for it, which she applied to helping with homework and giving tennis lessons; Jim taught at a boys' private school for twenty years; Harold was a popular TM teacher for as long as he could do it; and my sister Louise periodically held adjunct college teaching positions.

At two different times in my career I had interviewed for law school teaching jobs. I thought they might be the answer to my struggles with anxiety and identity. On the one hand, the subject matter was extremely practical—which, I hoped, meant no one would be able to claim I wasn't smart enough or emotionally strong enough to handle the "real world." But at the same time, I would be in academia, safely insulated from real-life consequences. Clients wouldn't be suing me for malpractice or complaining that a contract I'd negotiated had shortchanged them.

In both instances I withdrew my application after the final round of interviews. Although I did so for justifiable reasons— unwillingness to be geographically separate from Ed or to endure a two-hour commute with a newborn at home—I still wonder if there was another reason I backed out. Perhaps it was still less painful to be overwhelmed by anxiety than to acknowledge to myself that I couldn't handle the pressure of practicing law.

I'd like to say that the sixth-grade class went well because of my natural instincts for teaching and classroom management, but I'm certain it was because of the candy. A lesson on geography was actually an excuse to offer the students a taste of the different chocolates of the world.

I called Ed as soon as the first class was over.

"Ed, it was unbelievable."

"Yeah?" he asked tentatively, probably bracing himself for a story of disaster.

"I can't believe I am saying this, but it was fun. I really enjoyed teaching—seeing them get it was so exciting."

"That's great, Ame. I'm happy for you."

"Ed? I think I realized something . . ."

"What?"

"Um . . . well I . . ." I was stumbling more than usual, almost stalling, probably hoping to give the strange thought now bubbling up to consciousness time to sink back down to the depths.

"Tell me."

"I realized today that teaching doesn't have to be on some high intellectual level. It's the same act—the same feeling—as sharing something truly important. A gift. It felt so good. I mean, almost like loving them."

"That's so great," he repeated. "Maybe you should think about teaching."

"Elementary school?"

"Or middle or high school. I haven't heard you so excited about something in a long time."

"Oh God." I turned away from the cell phone in my hand and exhaled. As long as I practiced law, I could reassure myself that I was far more stable than my father. No matter how unjustified or irrational the equation, or how anxious the practice of law made me, wearing the label of "lawyer" was, for me, shorthand for "emotionally healthy." I brought the phone back up to my ear. "People would think it's so weird. Going from law to teaching kids. I would feel kind of stupid."

"Amy, if that's what you want to do, who cares?"

But of course I cared. Make a choice that practically screamed that I couldn't handle being a lawyer? That I was incapable, like my father, of holding a "real" job?

After the incident in New Haven and his hospitalization, my father had been employed only in the academic world: for a year as a college freshman English teacher and for about two years supervising the distribution of books to Bangladeshi libraries. Despite knowing that the original insult—"those who can, do; those who can't, teach"—was both unfair and untrue, I'd internalized a revised version based solely on my father's work experience, as I interpreted it: "Those who are emotionally secure, do; those who aren't, teach." And, even more threatening to my self-image, teaching at the primary or secondary levels might call into question not only my emotional security but also my intellectual ability; at least my father had managed to teach at the college level, even if only briefly.

I couldn't face it. But I also knew that my clinging to the law wasn't just the result of insecurity. It was that of a sniveling snob, desperately hanging on to some fictional self, a log in the open seas.

———

And yet I couldn't deny the genuine thrill I'd felt in the classroom. So, over the next two years, I secretly took graduate education courses and gradually tried on the idea of becoming a teacher.

By the time I decided to quit my law job to student teach full-time, I had developed just enough courage to stop hiding behind the law. The partners at my firm smiled and shook their heads condescendingly, fully confident that I would eventually return, either because I couldn't find a teaching job (after all, I was forty-eight) or because I'd tired of the public school teaching profession's lack of prestige.

It took me a while to figure out how to explain in cover letters and interviews why I'd changed careers. Like my insecure
inner snob, school administrators were incredulous that I would
leave the law for teaching. I wasn't always sure why they reacted
that way. Was teaching really that awful? Or did they hold the
law in higher esteem than their own profession? In any event, I
was eventually able to deflect their questions by responding,
with a laugh, "You know, it's only other lawyers who understand
my decision. They're all jealous." Which, in fact, was not much
of an exaggeration. If the public thinks that reining in adoles-
cents is difficult, they haven't dealt with clients raging over a
divorce or a real estate deal or a partnership agreement.

And although I was overwhelmed by every aspect of teaching, I could say for the first time in my life that I loved my job.
I'd finally reached a decision that felt like the first solid compo-
nent of an authentic identity. Having taken forty-eight years to
get there, I felt the relief of a stone-dragging Egyptian slave
who'd finally heaved her load onto the base of the pyramid.

———

My first year of full-time teaching, combined with the whirl-
wind of life with my eleven- and fourteen-year-old sons, was
exhausting but never once something I dreaded, as I had my law
jobs. By the end of January I was, however, counting the days
until my weeklong February break, when I could catch up on
sleep.

A week before the vacation, I heard Geanie's voice on the
answering machine and picked up.

"Hey, Geanie. How are you? How's the move going?"

I was certain she was calling to let me know when she and my father would be completing their move from Bronxville to their new apartment at Peconic Landing, an upscale retirement community at the end of Long Island's North Fork, which was about an hour's drive from my house. But her tone suggested a topic more serious than travel logistics.

"Amy, your father's really upset. He's very agitated about the move."

"Oh, I'm sorry. Is he okay?"

"Well, it's bad, Amy. I think he might hurt himself."

"*What?*" He hadn't been seriously depressed in years, and it had been a relief not to have to worry about him. Pinches of heat stung my cheeks, but any anger quickly dissolved into resignation. I was back on guard duty. I closed my eyes, cupped the mouthpiece with the heel of my hand, and slowly exhaled. I didn't ask Geanie how she knew he'd hurt himself. What he'd said or did. If I didn't know the details, I could create my own story, one that might not compel me to walk through that sludge of sadness.

"Yes," she said, "maybe even suicidal. I can't leave him alone. I've talked to Dr. Caldwell, and she agrees. She's found a really nice place near White Plains for him to stay while I make this move. I can't have him here and worry about him. It's too much."

"You mean a mental hospital or something?"

"Well, yes. It's small, very nice. He can get some help there."

"And his psychiatrist thinks he should go there?" I was wondering if (hoping that) Geanie was just overreacting. After all, moving would be stressful for anybody at their ages, Geanie at eighty-one and my father at eighty-six.

"Yes, absolutely. It's only for a couple of weeks or so, until I can get everything sorted out. Do you think you could pick him up when it's time for him to come out to Peconic Landing?"

"Yeah, of course, Geanie, of course." I couldn't argue with her. God forbid I convinced her to let him stay and he attempted suicide.

My jaw tightened. I did not want to be sucked into that vortex of worry and responsibility, but any thought of defiance was quickly extinguished by shame at my selfishness. Furthermore, it would be less painful for me to immediately assume guard duty than to disentangle the emotions engendered by my father's precarious mental state.

I might as well have pulled the master switch on prison floodlights, because almost instantaneously the buzzing that had just begun to reverberate in my chest whizzed out through my arms, down my torso, and into my legs so that even my fingers and toes were tingling.

———

During the next week I could only think about my father during the few moments of peace that teaching seventh grade and keeping up with my two teenage sons allowed. Making the six-hour round trip (under good conditions) to visit him would've been impossible, so I reassured myself that he was safe and I had a few weeks before having to face what might come next. And so, five days later, the first day of my vacation, I couldn't believe it when I heard my father's voice on the other end of the phone.

"Ame, honey. It's Dad. You've got to come pick me up. Now."

I squeezed the phone. He never issued demands. Requests, if ever made at all, were always couched in the most accommodating terms. I looked out at the falling snow, which had already left a foot on the ground.

"Oh God, Dad. Are you okay?"

"Ame. Please, honey. It's bad."

"Dad, is there snow up there? It's practically a blizzard here. The roads must be terrible."

"Please come, Ame."

I couldn't do it. I couldn't risk his or my safety in attempting the trip. I couldn't bear subjecting Ed to what surely would be a nightmare for him if I got stuck somewhere and needed his help. So, staring out at the snow, exhausted from a week of teaching, I gave myself one day to prepare for whatever might come.

"Dad. I can't. I'm really sorry. I promise I'll come as soon as the roads are clear."

"Tonight?"

"No, Dad. More like tomorrow morning, hopefully. They'll probably be okay by then."

———

The roads weren't great the next morning, but I made it there without too much difficulty. I turned onto a downhill driveway that led to a scattering of one-story, brownish-red brick buildings, their wooden shutters rimmed with snow. It looked like something between an institution and a residence. The waiting room was not inviting; its slightly shaggy carpet sported what was either a design of various shades of light brown or a number of stains, and its walls were lined with a haphazard mix of wooden, upholstered, and folding chairs. A woman sat behind a counter.

"I'm here to pick up my father, Harold Turner."

"Ohhh . . . hmmm . . . Yes, Mr. Turner," she said, nodding.

"Well, can I pick him up?"

We briefly discussed whether the facility's psychiatrist had agreed to release him, but I made it clear I was not leaving without him. As much as I wanted more time to myself, I could not leave him in such a shoddy-looking place, especially when he had been so uncharacteristically demanding. I reminded her that he hadn't been committed and could sign himself out.

Fortunately, she dropped the issue.

"First let me give you his medications." She handed me a large Ziploc bag that must have contained fifteen amber-colored plastic containers. She noticed my surprise. "And there's more," she said as she lifted another Ziploc bag onto the counter.

My father walked into the waiting room a few minutes later. He was carrying a small duffel bag and looked startled to see me. I grabbed his medications, signed the last few forms, and we walked out to the car.

———

As we drove up the hill to the exit, I saw three people walking in our direction, bundled up against the cold and waving enthusiastically. I slowed down. My father looked over at me with a smile before rolling down his window.

A boy, about sixteen, leaned in. A few strands of dark, greasy hair had escaped his wool cap and a small gold ring dangled from his runny nose. "Hey, Harold. Are you leaving? Are you getting to go home?"

"I am, Evan. I'm . . . getting . . . to . . . go . . . home," he said in a tone I knew well—the one he used whenever presented with a gift or a compliment or an unexpected pleasure, his happiness tempered by the silent recognition that others may not be so fortunate. "This is my daughter."

"Hey, that's great, Harold. Take it easy, man, okay? You're a good guy." The other two, a girl and a boy about the same age, leaned in to add their farewells. "Yeah, Harold. You're pretty cool. Good luck."

Although they would not have been able to see me, I nevertheless waited until we turned the corner before I jerked my head around toward my father. "Dad, *who* were *they?*"

"Well, Ame"—he paused for a beat before continuing—"some of the residents. This is basically a place for teenagers."

I couldn't believe Geanie and the psychiatrist had thought this institution was appropriate for my father. Facing the upheaval of moving and the prospect of once again entering a mental institution seemed more than enough for an eighty-six-year-old man to bear without him also having to deal with teenagers. I hoped that at least he'd been spared the awkwardness of having group therapy sessions with them. But I couldn't judge Geanie and his psychiatrist for their decision when I hadn't been willing to get involved; for all I knew, it was the best situation available on such short notice.

———

I didn't know what to expect from him when we got home. I had no idea whether I should try to play therapist and assess his mental condition or pretend he was on an ordinary visit. For the moment, I did what he might have done.

"How about some poetry, Dad?"

Peter and I were sitting on the couch. My father was across from us in the brown leather chair next to the fireplace.

I read some of Billy Collins's poetry out loud. Not my father's usual Keats or Auden or Frost. Under the circumstances, I thought we needed a lighter touch. I let Peter choose the poems. The first, "Another Reason Why I Don't Keep a Gun in the House," about having to listen to the continuous barking of a neighbor's dog, always made us laugh. His second choice, "On Turning Ten," seemed appropriate as well. It expressed the weight of sadness I first felt, at age four, as we drove home after waving to my father as he stood on the balcony at Lawrence Hospital.

———

The next day, after breakfast, my father and I sat in the living room and read to ourselves. I had almost forgotten he was there when I heard his voice.

"Ame, I'm not feeling well."

"Oh sorry, Dad."

"I have a pain in my stomach."

"Jeez, Dad. How long have you had it?"

"A couple of months, I think, maybe more. But now, honey, I think I better go to the emergency room. I'm sorry, Ame. Sorry to put you to the trouble."

I didn't question him. He had always been stoic when it came to physical discomfort. If he'd ever mentioned it to Geanie, he'd probably never acknowledged the pain.

And so the very day after I'd picked him up from the psychiatric facility, I took him to the local emergency room, where that evening he had surgery to remove a gangrenous gallbladder that the CAT scan tech told me, with some amazement, was the size of a grapefruit. With a difficult stay in the ICU followed by a stint on a regular floor, my father didn't get to Peconic Landing for a month.

21

CONTACT THROUGH
THE ETHER

ABOUT SIX MONTHS AFTER I'D FOUND THE NEWSPAPER
articles at the New York Public, I lay in bed with a terrible case
of bronchitis, searching my laptop for a photograph Peter had
asked for. I was paying little attention as I clicked through the
images—until a photo of Father Keating's letter to my mother
opened.

As I reread the letter, I realized what I should have thought
about long ago: Father Keating had saved my life as well as my
father's. What would have happened to me as the daughter of a
father who had chosen to die rather than to love his children?

A quick Google search revealed that I wouldn't be able to
thank him. He had left St. Mary's in 1976 and died in Washington, DC, in 2005 at the age of eighty. As I read his obituary, it
struck me again: What had prepared this man, at the age of thirty-
two, to save my father's life? What had he said to my father,
eleven years older and not religious in any way, to convince him
to climb back through that window? It couldn't have been years
of experience in the priesthood. According to the obituary, he
had been ordained in June of 1956, less than two years earlier.
And what experiences in his life had prepared him to write such

an insightful and compassionate letter to my mother, a perfect stranger?

Suddenly overwhelmed by gratitude for Father Keating's sensitivity and strength, and a dreaminess likely induced by having sipped NyQuil for an hour, I wrote to the prior of St. Mary's Church:

Dear Father Allen,

I feel compelled to write, but to whom I'm not sure, about the kindness of Father James D. Keating who served at St. Mary's Parish from 1956 to 1976. I am hoping that there is someone still at St. Mary's who knew him or of his work or if not, that others at St. Mary's would appreciate knowing that he is lovingly remembered for something he did fifty-five years ago.

I am a sixty-year-old married mother of two, an attorney turned schoolteacher.... How I wish I had thought to look him up [sooner] so that I could express my gratitude to him.

I have attached his letter to my mother because I don't think I can adequately express the sensitivity, generosity, and acceptance, which it conveyed. Though long ago I found a way to make peace with my father's lifelong illness, this beautiful expression of kindness and faith has become a touchstone for me. It must have been deeply comforting to my mother both during the ordeal and, as she kept it with her important personal correspondence until her death, for years after. That this letter continues to offer solace and love to me fifty-five years later is a testament to Father Keating's ministry for which I am profoundly grateful.

Thank you for reading this. If you know of someone else to whom my letter might be of interest, please share it.

With gratitude for Father Keating and the work of St. Mary's,

Amy Turner

I pressed send, releasing into the ether a prayer of sorts— one about as likely to reach anyone who knew Father Keating as it was to reach God.

———

When I opened my email the next day, I found a message from St. Mary's. I stared at it for a minute, thinking I couldn't possibly have received a reply, especially over Easter, the busiest weekend on the Christian calendar. But the email was an invitation to contact the head priest, who had known Father Keating.

I lay back against my pillow and closed my eyes. If I reached over and picked up the phone, I might in a matter of minutes receive the answers to my questions. What if Father Allen knew what my father had been thinking on that ledge? I couldn't bear the thought of hanging up and being left alone with the feeling that my father's story—in which mine was so bound up—was significant only for the pain and depression it had spawned in the rest of us. I needed a hint of courage, or redemption, or fun-

damental truth to also lie at the heart of my father's experience—a glimmer of hope amid the darkness Father Allen would
surely describe.

I couldn't do it. I told myself the head priest would be too
busy to speak with me. Better to wait until Easter was over,
maybe even another week. Surely the church would need time to
get back to handling administrative chores after such an important holy day.

Ed often asked me whether I'd called Father Allen yet, but
months went by and my answer was always no.

———

Then one day I finally worked up the nerve to call. Father Allen
was so gruff that one might have thought he was talking to a
telemarketer, not someone whom he had invited to call him. He
couldn't tell me much more than that he had known Father
Keating in Ohio, where he had lived after his stint at St. Mary's.
He was aware that Father Keating had worked with street youth
in New Haven and had been a prison chaplain. No, Father Keating had never mentioned the experience with my father.

Perhaps, I thought to myself, it had just been all in the day's
work of a priest.

Father Allen was even more curt when I reiterated my gratitude for Father Keating. I was disappointed. I had waited so long
to talk to him, and I'd worked up my courage in order to have
some closure. When I brushed my hurt aside, anger filled the
empty space. Couldn't he give me, a lapsed Episcopalian, a little
more grace for going out of my way to thank him for the work of
a Catholic priest when every day there was another revelation of

sexual abuse by Catholic priests that the church had attempted to cover up?

But I said nothing of the sort and began my goodbye.

As if reading my thoughts, he interrupted, "Hold on, wait a minute." Thirty seconds later, speaking to himself as much as to me, he said, "Yes, I thought so. I thought I was right. Today is the anniversary of Father Keating's death."

That was enough. Somehow I had reached Father Keating through the ether.

―――

Although I had confirmed the basic facts of my father's attempt and reached a dead end with Father Allen, I didn't have that sense of relief that comes with complete understanding.

Again, Ed suggested I just give it up. "I hate to see you so preoccupied," he would say gently. But I couldn't. If a fear of mental illness was my father's legacy to me, so was his oft-dispensed prescription: If something is upsetting you, "dig deep."

A few days after the call with Father Allen, I retrieved the Daily News article from the folder at the bottom of the stack on my desk and noticed what should have been obvious a year earlier when I had first seen it: the credit under the photograph on the front page of the Daily News was for the New Haven Register.

I could not believe I had missed it. My Google searches had turned up photographs of my father on the ledge in the International Herald Tribune, Paris edition, then on the front pages of the morning and evening editions of the tabloid New York Sun, now out of print for decades, but nothing in the New

Haven Register. I wondered if my dull-witted research had been some self-initiated form of the Somatic Experiencing technique of titration, allowing me to learn and see only what I could tolerate at the time.

But my subsequent research of the *New Haven Register* involved more frustration than titration. I located a citation to an article on the event, "Priest Prevents Suicide Leap from Fifth Floor of Hotel Taft," but the librarian at the New Haven Library couldn't access it for me.

After several weeks of phone tag and miscommunication, I was connected to another reference librarian who happened to be filling in that day. Unlike the other librarian, she sounded interested in the research. She promised to get back to me.

———

A few hours later on that gray and rainy February day, I was on my way to a restaurant to meet a friend for lunch, trudging with my head down to break the wind, when my phone rang.

It was the New Haven Public Library. I could bear the weather for this call.

"Amy? I found some things for you."

"Oh great, the article?"

"Yes, and more: an interview with Father Keating, and his obituary as well."

I hoped she hadn't heard my sudden exhale. It should have occurred to me to check for a local obituary, even if he had spent the last thirty years of his life elsewhere. I barely registered the rain cascading off my nose.

"This was your father who was . . . " She hesitated—to find a tactful way to describe the incident, I assumed. "Was involved at that situation at the hotel?"

She sounded so concerned I felt I should reassure her. "Yes, but you know, he went on to live a long life. Died when he was ninety. He was happy, fine. I just wanted to look into the family history."

"Well, I was interested myself because I knew Father Keating."

Cars were splashing through puddles, and the wind was interfering with the cell phone reception. Perhaps I hadn't heard her correctly. "Sorry, I'm not sure I heard what you said."

"I knew Father Keating. He was my Sunday school teacher at St. Mary's. He was such a wonderful man. A really good teacher. The kids all loved him. When we were older he ran a teen group that kids went to. He did get upset when kids started to have long hair and were against the war. He was conservative about that—Vietnam."

"Oh, thank you. I'm so glad to know that Father Keating was well loved."

"Yes, that he was. I'll mail the obituary and interview to you."

As I gave her my address, I decided not to request overnight delivery.

———

When the interview and articles arrived, I made myself breathe slowly and deeply. I also looked away after every few paragraphs, trying to stem the anxiety that rose each time I asked myself whether I would finally learn why my father climbed onto the ledge and then changed his mind.

The interview took place the day after the incident. According to Father Keating, he and the prior and another priest, Father Murphy, were walking across the New Haven Green when they heard some commotion and saw a crowd growing over by the Taft Hotel. The prior said they should go over to see if they could help. When they got there, they could see my father standing on the ledge and the fire ladders and circular net at the ready.

The prior told Father Murphy to stay on the sidewalk in case "last rites were needed" and asked Father Keating to accompany him upstairs. Once inside my father's room, and without explaining his choice, the prior asked Father Keating "to see what he could do."

Oh God, I thought. Fifty years later and I could hardly bear the thought of my father standing on the ledge and considering a jump. Yet this priest, in only seconds, was prepared for the worst. According to the interview, Father Keating's goal had been to keep my father talking and to discourage him from looking down.

A few seconds into their conversation, it was apparent that my father was less afraid of colliding with the pavement fifty feet below than of confronting what awaited him in the hotel room. My father "said," but I imagined he moaned, "If I come in there, the police will beat me up."

Father Keating "reassured him," saying, "I promise you, I will not let anything happen to you."

My father wasn't convinced. "Oh, what's the use," he said, "I'll spend the rest of my life in jail."

Father Keating urged him not to look down and kept talking.

Did he sense that my father, ever the gentleman, would defer to the rules of proper etiquette even when on the verge of suicide? Father Keating asked questions that required answers, which required replies, and then responses, a tether of words extending between them. According to the interview, at one point, my father, startled by a man who had stuck his head outside a nearby window, scared Father Keating by "hesitat[ing] for the moment and look[ing] toward the street below." As he looked down at the street, perhaps he was reminded once again of the appealing certainty that after a jump there would be no jail, no humiliation—a final blackout to his struggle with darkness.

Did my father notice the circular safety net and around it the faces of the firemen straining to hold it up at shoulder height—palms up, elbows out, eyes fixed—as they anticipated the potential location of my father's landing? Was at least one student in the crowd of hundreds who gathered picturing those Saturday morning cartoons where the rescuers frantically zigzag about, trying to position the net, as the hapless victim hilariously teeters in the opposite direction?

Father Keating spoke quickly, tightening the tether as fast as he could, "to relieve the tension of that episode."

"They won't take you to jail. I won't let them. I promise you that they will not do anything to you because of what you've done."

"But, if I don't go to jail," my father "said"—but I pictured him whimpering and wondered if it was at this point (as shown in one of the photos) that he clutched his forehead and covered his eyes, as if to shield himself from a sudden vision—"I'll spend the rest of my life in an insane asylum."

"Absolutely not. People can be cured of mental illness," Father Keating said, enunciating, I imagined, each word slowly and deliberately in an effort to eliminate or at least disguise any trace of doubt in his voice. That pledge would have been reassuring coming from any Catholic priest, but I wondered if Father Keating's physical bearing—his broad shoulders perhaps a reflection of his athletic career as a star high school football player and Navy boxing champion—was more comforting to my father, perhaps suggesting the strength to rescue him from jail or an asylum.

According to Father Keating, after fifteen minutes, "which seemed like fifteen years," my father stepped toward him, threw his arms around him, and allowed himself to be pulled into the hotel room. One man threw a coat over him (having spent twenty minutes outside, barefoot and pajama-clad, he was not just shivering from shock), another gave him a cigarette, and a third held out a cup of coffee, which he helped my father to sip from tentatively because he was "shaking too much" to hold the mug. I imagined him standing there with his neck outstretched, like a baby bird craning for food. Could he hear the crowd cheering below?

Inside the hotel room, as Father Keating had promised, there were no handcuffs, no rough stuff, no mean talk. My father was taken downstairs, and as he passed through the lobby to the hotel entrance and ambulance waiting outside, a UPI photographer snapped another picture. He was taken to the local hospital and later that night transported to New York Hospital, Westchester Division, where my mother met him. I remember her telling me that when she saw him for the first time he just stared at her, his eyes glassy and wide. He didn't recognize her.

As I finished the article, I wondered whether my father, lying in bed in the "asylum" that he'd so feared, ever thought of Father Keating's promise that he wouldn't spend his life there. But of what, exactly, had Father Keating assured him? If he wouldn't spend his entire life in an insane asylum, just how long would he have to stay? Even if he split the difference between his current age and, with some actuarial predictions, his age at death, did he worry he might spend another twenty years in the mental hospital?

22

STAYING CLOSE

EVEN AFTER READING THE INTERVIEW WITH FATHER
Keating, I still couldn't look at the photographs of my father on
the ledge for more than a moment at a time. Despite the precau-
tions I took before looking at the photographs—*take a deep
breath, shoulders down and back, pretend the man on the ledge is a
stranger*—I couldn't ignore the buzz that seemed to suck all the
oxygen from my chest. My body had its own timetable for this
venture, and it was not in any rush.

Every time I glanced at the images, I had a recurring
thought: *I was there.* With no warning, fifty-five years would
disappear faster than a camera's click. No time or space for clawing my way back to the present. *He could have jumped, and I
would have had a very different life.* Frozen in that frame, together
on the ledge—my father in utter despair, me in utter panic. I was
terrified by his vulnerability, and mine. If he'd jumped, what
would have happened to us? And how would we have lived with
our failure to save him?

But far more frightening, I suddenly realized, was the possibility that I couldn't have stopped myself either.

That was it. I wasn't just standing on the ledge with him . . . I
was him.

Looking at the shot of him climbing back to safety provided

only momentary relief. Before I'd seen those photographs, I could comfort myself with the distance and fantasies of power that imagination provided. I had barely, if at all, thought of his state of mind on that ledge. I'd seen the entire incident from years later, a vantage point that allowed me to focus only on areas of safety—his long life, for instance, and my confidence that I'd overcome any emotional ramifications of his suicide attempt. But the actual truth was on the ledge.

I was sure I'd resolved the psychological issues stemming from my childhood. By the time of the accident, at age fifty-seven, I'd had years of therapy—enough to consider myself qualified, as I once joked to a friend who was having a difficult time, to be her therapist's warm-up act. If I hadn't removed all the psychic residue of my father's attempted suicide and hospitalization, I could at least recognize its impact. I was far more self-aware than I'd been twenty-five years earlier, when I'd whirled into a weeks-long cyclone of fury after Ed announced he was taking a hiking vacation with some colleagues. When after a few therapy sessions I finally stopped hiding behind my anger, the truth became obvious to me: I'd been overwhelmed by the pain of my four-and-a-half-year-old self who'd felt abandoned thirty years earlier.

At this point in my life, a trip Ed might take with the guys wasn't likely to trigger any hurt feelings—and if they did, I understood their origin and certainly didn't act on them. But given my reaction to the photos, I had to admit that my father's attempt and hospitalization still governed me, like a vestigial organ that refused to stop pumping.

I could never force myself to sit with those newspaper photos long enough to fully understand what frightened me so much. I was reminded of those class photo days during my early teaching career when two fellow seventh-grade teachers and I would be charged with lining up seventy-five twelve-year-olds in height order. Our task entailed peeling apart best friends who, perfectly matched in every aspect but height, clung together as though magnetized by their chatter; finding the short boys who hid behind their tallest friends, hoping to avoid the humiliation of standing next to, ick, a girl; and convincing the tallest girls, pretzeled into Houdini-like contortions, to stand up straight and join, ick, the tall boys.

For the first three years, the process was excruciatingly loud and frustrating and took at least thirty unbearable minutes of shouting and maneuvering. But fifteen minutes into the fourth year's photo session, when I was on the verge of either huddling in a corner and sobbing or throwing the body nearest to me across the room, I was suddenly gifted with the laser-like focus of a first responder. I spotted the gleam of the gym teacher's whistle hanging beside the door across the room, and acted.

Stunned by the whistle's shriek, that year the students allowed themselves to be rearranged into perfect height order within seconds.

Now, I told myself to just blow the whistle, so to speak—to make myself stay with the photographs. But my breath quickened at the thought, and I stared out the window in search of a distraction. I wasn't ready to be stunned; whatever truths the photos held for me must still be too painful.

That week I mentioned to Isabella that I couldn't look at those photographs of my father for any length of time. Before I could begin psychoanalyzing myself, she steered the conversation to my physical sensations.

"I guess it's a buzzing in my chest first," I said. "Then I just need to get up and walk away."

"Well, it's understandable that you might have a strong physical reaction. It's been there a long time. With a mentally ill father and an alcoholic mother, you couldn't have felt safe even before your father went into the hospital. Do you remember much from those years? I think you told me once about a visit to Lawrence Hospital."

"Yes, I was four, so I was in nursery school at Sarah Lawrence. I loved it so much—the stone turret and all. But I couldn't go that much. I was sick a lot that year—the measles, mumps, other things."

"The year your father was in the hospital?"

I exhaled slowly. "Yes. Oh God. I can't believe I've never once thought about any physical connection between them— that my illnesses could've been related to my feelings about his absence. Maybe I was just so sad he was gone, or maybe I got sick because he was in the hospital. A way to stay close to him, somehow?"

———

I loved Sarah Lawrence nursery school, especially its sunlit room with its long, low, blond-wood tables upon which art supplies were always available. Apricot juice would never again taste so good to me as it did then, when our teachers' assistants, the

Sarah Lawrence "girls," would carefully pour it from a can into Dixie cups.

The French doors led to a stone patio; from there, it was a short run down the grassy hill to a playground shaded by a stand of tall pine, its ground covered with soft needles. At the far end of the play area was the formal entrance, a castle-like stone arch that announced to the public what I already knew: nursery school was magical.

But in December, less than a month after my father was hospitalized, I seemed to start to contract every childhood disease imaginable, and subsequently missed much of the school year. Although the reason for my "confinement" may have been as simple as an immune system unequipped to fight the viruses swirling around nursery school or, as I was starting to piece together now, sadness at my father's sudden disappearance, or a combination of both, it also occurs to me that this might have been my first attempt in a lifelong mission to stand guard against threats to his emotional stability. It wasn't my mother who'd been the first to assign me (and for that matter, all of her children) the role of protecting our father—my subconscious had already taken that on long before she started cautioning us not to get him upset or angry. In my childhood thinking, if it was considered normal for a child to be sick enough to be kept in bed and isolated from everyone else for months, wouldn't it also be considered normal for my father to be as well? If I was in bed too, there was no need for him to feel remorse about his absence.

———

If I *was* trying to reassure my father by staying in bed, it was a Herculean effort. First I had the German measles. Then the mumps developed. Then the measles and the chicken pox appeared simultaneously. How Dr. Neuhardt could tell that the red splotches all over my body reflected two distinct diseases is a mystery. But he got to know me pretty well, as he seemed to be at our house every week.

Tall and heavyset, Dr. Neuhardt would climb the front stairs to my parents' bedroom, where I was moved for his visits, and sit on the edge of the bed. His weight caused me to roll toward him, giving me a closer view of his black leather satchel on the floor.

Nowadays all but a tired prop, back then the bag may as well have been a snarling dog crouching at his master's feet, just waiting for the command to attack. I would lie there praying that the command wouldn't come, that the needles and droppers would stay at bay. When a reach for the bag produced only a stethoscope, I breathed a sigh of relief. But eventually the drops would be unleashed.

In between more serious diseases, I had piercing ear infections that required me to lie still as Dr. Neuhardt dispensed warm liquid into my ears. Each drop hurt as it slowly made its way down the canal. And just as it reached its destination (I could always tell, because that was when it hurt the most), Dr. Neuhardt would release another. Eventually, like a backed-up sink, my ear would gurgle up the drops; by the fourth or fifth, it seemed that they would never go down. But when it was finally over, the worst possible news for me (and, God knows, my mother, as I was probably screaming and crying the entire time) was that I had a double ear infection. "Roll over, Amy. Other ear, please," Dr. Neuhardt would say—with some sympathy, but also in a tone serious enough to eliminate any hope for negotiation, which at that stage of my childhood would have been attempted by relentless whining.

According to my mother, my fevers often led to deliriums. I remember screaming for her to get Harold and Jimmy away from me. As she hurried into my room, she assured me that my brothers were downstairs. "See, Amy?" she said, quickly pulling back the window curtain to admit the afternoon sunlight. "They're not here. It was probably only a fly you heard." I wasn't so sure about that, but her palm on my forehead, which must have been burning, cooled and comforted.

One of my strongest memories from this time is of the handwritten letters my father sent to each of my siblings and me. They represented another fundamental tenet of his philosophy—that words could heal. Whether you found them through reading or writing or speaking to a therapist, verbal expression born of unearthing the truth (and the deeper the dig, the better) was the greatest good. And his words did heal, at least during the time it took to recognize my name on the envelope, tear open the flap, and listen as my mother read the letter aloud.

The first letter I received was dated December 30, 1957, about six weeks after the suicide attempt. He explained what New Year's was: "It's the last night of this year, 1957—so the next day everyone will be saying 'Happy New Year' to each other, but I'd like to say it right now to you."

And what had he been thinking this New Year would bring *to him*? Recovery? I doubt he had had enough treatment by then to be so optimistic.

Despite all that he must have been pondering as 1958 began, his letters to me always contained humor—mostly for my benefit, I'm sure, but perhaps also for my mother, who would visit him on Sundays, often bringing gifts that we children had made for him.

A week after his first letter, he wrote, "I loved your 'creation,' which I took to be an animal, and therefore is now my pet."

By February he must have been feeling better, because he started including illustrations in his letters to me—which meant I could read them by myself. And I did, over and over. I loved to "read" my brothers' letters, as well. For Harold, my father drew three illustrations to accompany the following riddle: "1-a'lama is a priest, 2-a'llama is an animal, and 3-a'larma is a fire."

My favorite letter arrived just after the appearance of the red, pus-filled pimples of chicken pox. There I was, outlined in blue pen, lying in bed with medicine bottles clustered on the night table next to me; ink pox dotting my face; my eyes closed in two upside-down crescents; my mouth, one line curved down slightly, in less of a frown than the pursing of lips against a rising sob.

I loved that picture, and the letter—bearing the creases, tears, and stains of repeated reading—shows it. I don't think my father knew (or, under the circumstances, would have remembered if told) that my favorite book at the time was Ludwig Bemelmans's *Madeline*. I loved hearing about the twelve girls who lived in the care of the firm but loving Miss Clavell. For me, the best part was when Madeline was rushed to the hospital for an emergency appendectomy. She appeared on the page, simply drawn, sick and in bed, just like me (and my father too?).

And for Madeline and me both, a happy ending. When the eleven girls visited, Madeline stood on her hospital bed before them, proudly lifting her shirt to reveal her surgical scar. On the back of my father's letter I stood equally triumphant and tall, the ink curve of my mouth turned up in a broad smile, a small circle, labeled "nurse's graduation pin," shining on my uniform. And in the next picture, like I imagined my heroine Madeline might have done, I was jumping on my sickbed, my arms waving gleefully.

That year, whether sad or sick or both, I could always find comfort in *Madeline* and my father's letters, for—all the remedies in Dr. Neuhardt's bag notwithstanding—they offered the essential element of healing, the certainty that no matter how many times I opened the envelope or turned the book's pages, the exact same words would always be there. I know why I saved those letters through myriad moves and floods and other upheavals of adult life: they represented the last time my father knew me well enough to give me exactly what I needed.

23

LISTENING TO MY FATHER

THROUGH THE INTERVIEW WITH FATHER KEATING, I had gotten close enough to the ledge to practically hear his conversation with my father—but as happens with many research projects, it looked like the question most important to me might forever go unanswered. If Father Keating had known why my father had changed his mind, he hadn't said so, and my father wasn't alive to ask. But it suddenly occurred to me—as if I was titrating once again—that another conversation might hold the answer.

Jim had recorded a lengthy interview of our father for a graduate school paper on the Lawrence Hospital strike, which had occurred about seven years after the Taft Hotel incident. My father would have turned one hundred on his upcoming birthday in August of 2014. I suggested to Jim that, in light of this important birthday, it might be interesting to hear our father's voice again. I didn't tell him what I was looking for. I didn't want to discuss it. Perhaps my mother's iron curtain on this topic still had a hold on me.

Jim said he'd look through the tapes.

He called back sooner than I expected.

"I found one that is probably the most interesting, but"—he cautioned in a tone that suggested I should prepare myself for something upsetting—"it is very personal, Ame, very personal."

Jim transferred the tape to a CD for me, and when it arrived it was lovely to hear my father's voice. I'd almost forgotten how much kindness it conveyed. As I listened to him describe his experiences at Yale and at early jobs, I was struck by his honesty. He could have easily rationalized his less-than-flattering conduct by taking advantage of hindsight, but he did not.

As he moved through the 1940s and talked about going to an analyst in the 1950s, I began to steel myself. We were approaching 1957. His voice was slowing. I pictured him looking down, his eyes briefly closed, and then looking up at Jim with that familiar smile—the one that, despite the gleam in his eyes, conveyed not just his sadness but a recognition of others' suffering as well—as he said, "Well, then you know 1957, Jim, that was the darkest period of my life."

If I hadn't been so anxious, I would have considered what followed a farce: the CD stopped abruptly.

I checked the machine. Certainly something was stuck. I played with it, jostled it, took it out and reinserted it at least ten times. I'm embarrassed to admit I even turned it over and tried to play the other side. Then I tried it on my car's CD player. It stopped at the same place. *What?*

I told Jim that the CD seemed to stop abruptly at forty-five minutes even though he had said it was a ninety-minute interview. Jim found that hard to believe but had the same problem when he played it. I received two more copies over the next three months, and each one stopped at that "darkest period." My father's image frozen on that ledge; now his voice silenced as well.

Then Jim called to say he had finally found a competent recording company and that the corrected CD should arrive in a week.

I inserted the new disk and cued it to fifteen minutes before he mentioned 1957. I needed time to prepare. I listened to him talk about analysis, "all those defeats and failures," and of waking up in the Coast Guard and not being able to face the day. "We're getting into a very personal area, Jim. Well, then you know 1957, Jim, that was the darkest period of my life."

I steeled myself. The repaired CD picked up where the last had ended: "1957—I was in no condition to take on the responsibility of being a husband, and I guess I've been grateful I didn't do any worse as a father than I did." And that was it. He moved on to politics.

I gasped. My insides jolted, triggering a sudden sensation of whiplash. Although my mouth was half-open, I held my breath for a second, as if the circulating oxygen might help dispel my disbelief. My two-year search, albeit a fitful and inexpert one, had yielded nothing. Ed was the only other person who knew about it and would be supportive whatever the result, yet I was still embarrassed. It felt like the gods (or even my father, though he would never be unkind) had played a cosmic practical joke on me and then leaned in close and crowed, "Fake out!" My cheeks burned, but I smiled at the thought and took a few slow breaths.

I lay back, my head against the pillow, and closed my eyes. I would never know why my father had made the decision not to jump. But even in my disappointment, I could appreciate the irony. It was his story to tell, not mine.

24

THE PATIO CURE

DURING THE SUMMER OF 2014, FOUR MONTHS AFTER listening to my father's interview, I was outside on our deck, walking toward the French doors, as I'd done a million times before, when the photograph of my father on the ledge flashed in my mind so unexpectedly and rapidly that I thought I heard a camera click. I froze; noticing the white gutter pipe to my left, I considered touching it for support.

Instead, I closed my eyes. Suddenly, the insides of my eyelids burned. I swallowed some air, hoping it would prevent a cry, but a fugitive tear squeezed through the outside corner of my right eye and grazed my ear as it slid over my cheekbone. As my attention returned to my eyes, I realized I'd been observing physical sensations without associating them with any emotions or memories—the "story," as Isabella referred to them. In her office, her gentle reminders were sufficient to bring me back to my body, but on my own, I invariably tended to explore the psychological, a reflex born out of my many years in therapy (and from the fact that, since for most of my life my only interest in my body had been whether it was thin enough—which was rarely—monitoring my mind, whatever its state, was almost always less fraught for me).

Today, however, I continued scanning my body, following
the energy as it slowly descended along a familiar path, through
my head and into the fight-or-flight tension in my left shoulder,
the thickness in my chest, and the hollow of my palms. Then, as
though I were riding in an out-of-control elevator, I was suddenly
plunging downward. My stomach seemed to ricochet off my
Adam's apple, my heart pummeled my chest, and in an instant
my pelvis felt a jolt.

I resisted the impulse to open my eyes. The weight sank into
the deepest regions of my abdomen and spread outward to my
hips. I was reminded of the time Isabella had placed yoga weights,
small pillowcases filled with sand, right at those joints—to give
me, she said, a feeling of grounding. But this ballast, internal and
much heavier, resembled something else as well: that physical sensation that signals we've made the right decision or uncovered a
truth. But I'd done neither . . . yet.

I blinked at the sunlight as though awakening from a nap. I
knew the experience couldn't have lasted more than fifteen seconds, but I glanced around nevertheless, just to make sure that
nothing had changed. I was relieved to see that the dog still slept
under the table, the purple flowers still resisted the breeze, the
aroma of coffee still wafted from my mug. I was also relieved that
no one had seen me—which was absurd, since there had been
nothing to see. I hadn't even moved. Yet I did feel different. Transformation is too big a word, but I quickly looked at my reflection
in a window just to make sure I hadn't sprouted cockroach wings.

I replayed the experience in my head. As I recalled the jolt,
that sense of grounding, I understood all at once what the ledge
meant to me, why I'd been so afraid of those photographs. I
looked down, closed my eyes, and shook my head slowly, a

twinge of amusement and embarrassment that it had taken me so long to arrive at such a simple truth: *I was born on that ledge.* Not the "I" of my body, of course, which had entered the world four and a half years earlier, but the "I" of my *self.* I had internalized—at such an early age—my parents' struggles with themselves and each other so completely that I had actually embodied them.

———

It took a few hours before the slow but unstoppable sludge of depression worked its way into my bloodstream. Whenever I allowed myself to identify with my father's vulnerability, as I had on the patio, I'd eventually hear my mother's voice, thick with disdain, ricocheting around my brain: "He's sick, Amy, he can't handle it."

Pathetic is what she meant but never said—and as much as I tried to lower the volume, I never could. Now, angry, frustrated, and filled with self-loathing at my inability to silence her and empathize with my father, I felt a state of hopelessness, just as I had as a child who was unable to save her parents; the feeling was so familiar to me, in fact, that it almost comforted. Any power I sensed as a separate individual had been illusory, based on a child's desperate but mistaken belief that she could save her parents. There had never been enough space for an authentically independent self to take root.

I finally understood—no, actually felt in my body—the nature of my identity, but that understanding revealed another undeniable truth: I had spent fifty-five years in a mental prison of my own construction, and if I hadn't clanged the door open yet, I doubted anything could cause me to do it now.

———

I hadn't felt so utterly defeated in over ten years, since the Christmas after my mother died—"situational," my therapist called it. The feeling didn't lift the next day, or the next.

I told myself this was the effect of weaning off my tension headache medication, but my neurologist disagreed. It was summer. I could swim in the ocean off a pristine beach. Ninety-nine percent of the world would be happy to live where I did.

But neither logic nor the environment had any influence. In the mornings, I'd be lucky to have two neutral thoughts about the day's possibilities before full wakefulness brought with it an awareness of the slab lying on my chest, the pressure in my head, that familiar and unbearable weight of being myself. And on particularly bad days, as I heaved myself up to go to the bathroom, I was already crying before I picked up my toothbrush.

I was surprised when my therapist rather than her machine answered the phone. I had hoped to leave a message, a "feeling kind of depressed, not an emergency but probably would be good to come in" kind of thing, long enough to get the message across but brief enough not to trigger tears. Later I thought of the irony of making an appointment to discuss depression but not wanting to appear weak by crying over the phone. An internal struggle over the correct response to vulnerability: reveal even the most painful, my father would no doubt suggest; "just *do something*," my mother would snap with evident disgust. I compromised by briefly describing how I was feeling and dropping my voice an octave to squelch a sob. I made an appointment for the following week.

The next morning I lay back on one of the two chaises on our deck and looked around absently. On the table next to me sat that morning's third mug of coffee, which I'd hoped would elevate my mood enough for me to fake it through the afternoon. So far, it had produced only a tinge of nausea and heartburn.

From a distance, the white vinyl chaise, streaked with black mold, had a zebra-like quality. I wondered if zebras ever drank at swamps, for our small pool was beginning to resemble one. Through a confluence of circumstances that felt like a conspiracy between nature (a pine tree bent over by the winter's heavy snow had, until its recent and miraculous resurrection, prevented the removal of the pool cover) and our pool guy (who had been distracted for months by an ongoing divorce), it was mid-July and the pool had not yet been opened. The partially folded-back pool cover revealed a four-foot-deep, blackish-green lagoon. I looked away, but not quickly enough to avoid a wave of queasiness.

The view toward the house was only slightly more palatable. I recalled the pride I'd felt in choosing what turned out to be the perfect color for the doors and trim, a rich slate that complemented the light gray of the rest of the house. But we had completed that paint job more than ten years earlier, and now the French doors that opened to the deck were not only peeling but also bore the grooves left by our Labrador Veda's scratching. (Just then, she nosed her way through the flap of screen she'd torn away from the doorframe to join me outside.)

Ed and I, too, had abused those doors. When we discovered that Veda could open the front door by jumping up and bringing her paw down on the levered handle, we'd had to lock it. We'd never gotten around to replacing the handle, so every day, no matter how harsh the weather, we passed through a gate in the picket fence, climbed onto the deck, and entered the house through these deteriorating French doors.

I continued my inspection. The picket fence matched the chaises: originally white but by now blackened in places with areas of mold and exposed wood. Two of the pickets were missing; another, its top having split off, resembled a medieval weapon; and another, its bottom having decayed unevenly, had a snaggletooth look.

Totally submerged in the funk of my surroundings, I didn't hear my friend Margaret arrive until the picket fence gate clattered almost directly in front of me. We had a plan to meet at my house and then spend the day together at the beach. She glanced at the pool and then removed her sunglasses and half smiled at me, her eyebrows raised expectantly. The silent question a visitor poses to a sick friend: *How ARE you?*

Her inquiry about *me*, prompted as it was by the condition of our surroundings, was both question and answer. I laughed for the first time in days.

"Oh, Margaret, I can't believe I'm laughing. I was just lying here staring at this god-awful mess. I swear, as soon as you arrived, I realized this place is a manifestation of my mental state. I have been so depressed."

"Depressed? Oh, I'm so sorry. You should've called me."

"I haven't been able to move. Like the sludge in that pool."

"Well, let's start with that," Margaret said with a trace of self-mocking authority.

"I have lived like this for ages, but I'd never really seen it before. Look over there." I pointed to the ripped screens. "I can't do it anymore."

"Really—for ages?"

I was living like Pigpen, I realized. I pictured myself walking around with some squiggly lines above my head, like I had to be surrounded by confusion, a big, disordered mess, to feel comfortable. I looked up at Margaret, who was scanning the deck, no doubt redecorating it in her mind.

"Well, if you want to change it, just tell Ed."

"I can't. He's the one who's working. Money's a little tight. He'll get annoyed that I'm even asking."

"Amy, Ed loves you. He just wants to make you happy."

Of course I knew that. Ed had made many sacrifices for me, willingly and even happily, over the years. Yet telling him I wanted to fix a few things around the house seemed for some reason more daunting than telling him I wanted to quit my attorney job so that I could student teach for six months without earning any income. I wiped tears from my cheeks.

"I cannot believe I'm saying this," I confessed. "*But I am afraid to ask him.* I feel like some fifties housewife."

Maybe I didn't want to ask him. Maybe I just wanted to stay stuck. Stay as helpless as I'd felt as a child who, no matter how hard she had tried or hoped, could not save her parents. And worse than being futile, the attempts were risky. Say or do the wrong thing, and somebody might jump or drink.

"If it will help you with your depression just a little, I'm sure he wouldn't be annoyed."

"Yeah, and that's even more depressing. How superficial can I possibly be if some home improvement will cure my depression?"

During dinner I nodded patiently and *uh-huh*-ed in the right places as Ed catalogued the day's frustrations, from work to politics to incompetent drivers. I was embarrassed by my growing anxiety and hoped my face wasn't reddening. I'd been married to Ed for thirty-three years. Why was I acting like a wife on *Mad Men*?

I waited until I thought he'd exhausted his capacity for complaining.

"Umm, Ed. I need to say something . . ."

"Okay, well, say it then," he said, his voice carrying a trace of singsong. He turned away from me to shoo the cat off the table.

"No, I mean . . . this is difficult, I . . ."

"Oh." He sat up and looked at me.

"I can't . . . can't . . . stand it. Not another second. I don't know what's come over me. I was outside today lying on one of those chaises, and I couldn't bear it. It's so disgusting. Umm . . . I think it's really adding to my depression."

"What? The deck and the pool?" He leaned toward me across the table, his voice rising with incredulity and a twinge of defensiveness. "Adding to your depression?" He must have noticed the heat rising to my cheeks. He sat back, took a sip from his wineglass, and smoothed his tone. "It's been like that for a long time before you were depressed. It's never bothered you. I don't even notice it anymore."

"I know, I know." I looked down and closed my eyes. Suddenly, I felt like I was drifting out to sea on an island of calved ice. I could not believe that I was struggling to get the words out. "I can't explain it, Ed. It's just important."

"We don't really have much . . ." But Ed let his voice trail off before he said, "money." He looked up at me, nodded gently, and said, "Okay, okay. If you think it'll make you feel better. I'll text Besim."

Besim, deeply grateful to Ed for having hired him several years ago as a newly arrived and undocumented immigrant from Kosovo, was at our house the next morning at 11:00 a.m. I wondered if he was a mirage, a product of my wishful thinking, until his assistant came around the corner. I knew I lacked the power to manifest two men.

Besim took a small yellow notepad from his back pocket and followed me around as I pointed out the work to be done. Ed and I left the next day for Massachusetts, where we planned to spend a long weekend in a cabin deep in the woods in celebration of our thirty-third wedding anniversary.

———

If Besim's appearance less than twelve hours after Ed texted him had seemed like an illusion, then the sparkling turquoise pool, freshly painted doors, intact screens, and new fence still damp with white paint that greeted us upon our return was surely a hallucination. I opened my mouth to laugh but was too dumbstruck to make a sound. I stood there, my mouth frozen in a gaping grin.

Ed started mumbling, alternating between "I can't believe it" and "Oh my God."

"I don't even know what to say," I said. "I even feel so much lighter . . . freer . . . like some crane pulled me out of quicksand." I was stunned as much by what I was seeing as what I felt. Like all my arteries and veins had been unclogged at once and my blood could flow in a way it never had before. I felt a whoosh of air, like a heavy metal prison door had opened.

"Leave it to me," Ed said, smiling devilishly and twitching his eyebrows three times, Groucho-like.

"Yeah, as long as someone points it out to you first," I said, laughing.

———

The next morning, I sat in Barbara's small waiting area—I'd now been seeing her for therapy, on and off, for fifteen years—and pondered what to say about the patio transformation.

Barbara opened the door with her characteristic warmth and enthusiasm, and I forced myself to maintain eye contact until she had safely curled herself into her leather chair.

I sat on the white couch across from her, between us a small table on which sat her thick black-leather appointment book and all-important clock. After our phone conversation, she must have expected me to slump down into the couch and sigh between sobs, but I was sitting up straight, even leaning forward a little.

"Well," I humphed, a sheepish smile creeping across my face, "I've had the patio cure."

Barbara laughed. "And *what* is the patio cure?"

"Well . . ." I explained how transforming the deck had changed everything, how I could feel my depression just lift as soon as we got back and the work was done. "It seems so absurd," I finished, "but I knew that patio was *me*, somehow."

"Can you explain that a little more?"

"I've just been stuck. Like . . ." I clutched my hands together in a silent clap, my right thumb pinning my left, the other fingers of my right hand pressing against the back of my left—the position that makes a slight sucking sound when you pull your hands apart. And then, to demonstrate the force of the squeeze, I reversed my hands, left over right. The irony wasn't lost on me: I'd gone to therapy to find some words, but all I could do was move my body.

"Hmm . . . How did the depression start?"

"Remember how I've been struggling with looking at the pictures of my father on the ledge? Well, last week I suddenly flashed on a photograph of him—with the fire ladders—and had this weird sense I was born on that ledge. It was liberating at first, but by that night I was totally depressed."

"Why couldn't you sustain that liberation?"

I looked down. "It's related to what I'm doing with my hands. It just feels like who I am—like I'm squeezed inside this clap, no way for a *me* to emerge. And somehow it's all on that ledge."

"Yes, but of course, your identity developed as you got older—"

"*No, that's just it.*" My breath stuttered. "My identity *didn't develop* after that. That *was* my identity. Right there on that ledge. Built on the fear of vulnerability. And so I was forever stuck."

I clasped and reclasped my hands again. I talked for a long time, as if in a trance. I looked over at Barbara, but I couldn't quite gauge her response. She was squinting, as though mulling over something, but in the smile emerging on her face there was the slightest hint of something—a realization (or diagnosis?)—occurring to her. It made me nervous.

"Did that make any sense?" I asked when I was done.

She hesitated for a moment. What had I said? *Patio cure?* Was I crazy? Or terminally superficial?

"Well . . . there is a term for what you're describing . . ."

"Really? What?"

"Undifferentiated ego mass."

"What?" I burst out laughing and threw myself against the cushions beside me, and almost ended up lying on my side. "Mass? I am picturing some disgusting cyst, like the one my gynecologist removed from my ovary and thought I'd like to see!"

I laughed out of surprise, but out of relief as well. Although I'd never before heard the term, it did seem accurate in some onomatopoeic kind of way: it sounded as tangled up as the actual state of mind it was describing.

"Yes. It's exactly what you're talking about. A differentiated ego never really forms because the child is so emotionally fused with the parents. In fact, the entire family can be stuck in sort of an emotional oneness."

"Barbara, all this time I'd convinced myself I had grown, had separated from my parents—becoming a teacher, trying to be a stable parent, having a fairly healthy marriage. And my parents have been dead for over ten years."

"Yes, Amy, those steps were progress and they weren't easy for you . . ."

"Yeah, but I think they were disguises, somehow. Those decisions were just a big, complicated mess of responses to my parents. That's why I never researched the ledge. That's why I couldn't look at the photograph once I'd found it. I had to face that after fifty years I was still—despite all my efforts—stuck there."

"But you did see it. Some people never do."

"Well, now if I feel the sludge rising, I'll know it's that undifferentiated ego mass sucking me in, and I won't get lost in it. Maybe it's time to build an ego, an identity. Like what most people do as children, hopefully."

Barbara's smile widened.

"I guess I have a few pieces in place," I said. "But I wonder who I'll be?"

———

Later that summer I decided to search "Harold Turner and the Taft Hotel 1957" one more time, just in case I'd yet again overlooked some obvious source. I wouldn't have been surprised if another newspaper had popped up. But when I saw a link to eBay titled, "1957 Press Photo New Haven, Conn. Rescue of Harold Turner on Ledge of Hotel" in "Collectibles, Photographic Images," I blinked. *For sale?*

The screen went black as it retrieved the site and then filled with an enlarged close-up of the three-paneled sequence of my father on the ledge, Father Keating in the window beside him, showing details that couldn't be detected in the grainy newspaper photos. I could see their faces, the folds in their clothing. My father's eye sockets were hollow, dark holes where his eyes should have been. His pajamas, partially tucked in, draped over his waist and ankles. His right sleeve hung down, hiding his hand.

Father Keating's face appeared slightly round, perhaps only in contrast to the gauntness of my father's cheeks. His skin looked smooth to the touch, as though his years in the priesthood had shielded him from some of life's anguish. The white of his priest's collar matched the hint of a shirt cuff visible at the edge of his black cassock.

In the second shot, my father was clutching his face with his right hand and extending his left arm against the building to maintain his balance. The smallest toes and outermost edge of his left foot were hanging off the ledge.

I walked over to our French doors. Just a few feet outside, perched at the end of an oak branch, a brilliant red cardinal stood impassively, its beak slightly upturned into the wind. Standing guard, I thought to myself. I looked beyond, to the blue patches outlined by the leafy branches. I thought of that moment when the truck was pulled off me and, lying on the pavement, I looked up to see the trees growing so impossibly tall in front of me and was suddenly awash in gratitude and love.

I returned to the image of my father on the ledge. I noticed that the buzzing in my chest, the familiar harbinger of the anxiety and worry to follow, was gone. Instead, I felt a sense of lightness, of a space opening within me, a sensation that until then I'd only felt lying on Isabella's treatment table. Although she'd said that one day I would integrate that internal distance so fully that it would affect how I responded to stress, I'd doubted that would happen for me. But now even the finest hairs on my body seemed to relax, as though they'd been graced by a gentle wind.

25

"EXTRA, EXTRA"

IN THE FALL OF 2015, A FEW WEEKS AFTER SCHOOL started, I was googling social studies resources for my classes when I came across a newspaper archive I'd never seen before. Looking for a distraction and almost without thought, I entered a search, "Harold Turner, 1957, New Haven." The search icon's rotation slowed to a cockeyed wobble—surely, I thought, the sign of an imminent error message—but moments later, the results filled three screens. I closed my eyes and exhaled with a humph that sounded, I realized, like my mother. If she had known about this extensive coverage, our family lore would surely have included it.

I appreciated the absurdity. I had panicked at the New York Public Library upon first sight of the *Daily News* article and for months afterward tried to avoid looking at it. But fifty years ago, big-city and small-town newspaper editors alike had decided— presumably on deadline and in a matter of minutes—that their readers wouldn't want to miss this story.

Having finally gained enough emotional distance (or maybe differentiation?), I could now handle what I was seeing in front of me.

It took only a few seconds of scrolling for me to realize how far-flung these newspapers were. The images of my father had appeared in more than eighty newspapers in a total of thirty-one states across the country, including one in Paris. Their circulations were just as wide-ranging, from large cities like Los Angeles, Detroit, Philadelphia, and New York to small towns such as Freeport, Illinois; Zanesville, Ohio; Ottawa, Kansas; and Kane, Pennsylvania.

As each image opened, my heartbeat stuttered only slightly; I no longer needed to titrate my exposure. From the photo attributions, I could tell that the different images had something to do with the particular wire services to which the newspapers subscribed, but even so, editors made changes to those photos provided. The Bridgeport, Connecticut, paper showed a tall ladder reaching up the side of the hotel's exterior where my father stood on a ledge against the building's facade. It emphasized "height" and the associated "danger." The photo in the North Dakota paper showed him clinging to the side of the building on a "precariously narrow" ledge. You couldn't tell how high off the ground he was, but he was clearly in an unstable position. The Freeport, Illinois, paper printed the three-photo triptych that I'd seen on eBay that showed my father standing on the ledge, then talking to Father Keating, and finally climbing back into the "safety" of the hotel.

As almost half of the newspapers were subscribers to the Associated Press and thus published variations of the same photos, eventually I was lulled into a half daze by the mechanical routine of click, enlarge, print. But when the International Soundphoto image filled my screen, I flinched. Steeply angled upward, the shot captures my father looking down at the sidewalk and seemingly directly into the camera, giving the viewers of 1957—and me—the sense of making eye contact with him as he makes his life-or-death decision. Despite the graininess and distance of the image, viewers could plainly see my father's agony and fear—his skull-like black eyes, his slightly opened mouth—and, if only for a moment, might have felt, as I did, the instinct to rescue him. I felt a wave of sorrow and guilt—for being incapable of helping him in 1957 or right then, as I returned my father's imploring stare—wash over me. Yet those feelings left nothing in their wake as I moved on to the next photo.

———

It was obvious why I was interested in the photos, but now I wondered what editors saw in the photos that had prompted such wide coverage.

Perhaps it was what was happening in America in 1957 that made the image of my father standing alone on a ledge in a moment of life-or-death decision-making so compelling. The news stories that dominated the headlines during the first eleven months of 1957 could certainly have generated feelings of fear, despair, and vulnerability. Front pages reported on civil rights protests, the launch of Sputnik, and the inception of the space race; hearings of the House Un-American Activities Committee (HUAC); a flu pandemic in which 70,000 Americans died; the opening of the first nuclear power plant in the US; escalating violence in Vietnam; and, of course, the Cold War between the USSR and the US, with Eisenhower and Khrushchev at the controls. It struck me that the front page of the November 14, 1957, *Daily News* captured both the private and public angst of the time. The photos of my father standing on the ledge appear just below the words *"MUST SPEND TO ARM, SAYS IKE – Cites 'Red Danger to Free Men'"*—which headline a story on the burgeoning arms race between the US and USSR.

Many readers, whether or not they would admit it, might have been curious about (if not personally impacted by) suicide. Although at that time the public, including my family, generally considered suicide a taboo subject, it ranked among the ten most common causes of death in close to half of US states. Everyone recognizes at some point, if only fleetingly and privately, that we can end our lives at any time. The thought might occur in a moment of despair, or possibly as a matter of instinct when, standing at a great height, we experience that shocking impulse to jump, whether or not we ever feel compelled to act on it. Those of us who can tolerate the discomfort might recognize that we are always on the ledge, that each morning we decide (to the extent it is within our control) whether to go on living that day.

The photographs of my father, offering an intimate view of his agonizing decision-making, would allow others to consider suicide openly and from a vantage point of relative emotional safety: they didn't know him, and the incident ended "happily."

Perhaps cultural anxieties of the time might also have contributed to the images' appeal. Existentialist thought— with its view that we live in an indifferent and absurd universe, and, without a god, must "decide for ourselves the meaning of our existence"—had reached the mainstream. Samuel Beckett's *Waiting for Godot*, published in 1952, first produced in 1953, and appearing on Broadway for the first time in 1956, had existentialist themes, focusing on two men waiting for an individual (or a salvation) that never arrives.

We are alone in an irrational universe—alone on a ledge, so to speak. Although some might have viewed this freedom as liberating, others—especially in small-town America, where tradition and religion have always had their strongest hold—could have seen it as terrifying.

In that era, close to half of all Americans (including my family) attended church on a regular basis. Newspaper editors had reason, then, to expect the story of a priest saving a man to be of great interest to their readers, providing them with a newspaper-reading experience as reassuring as it was rare: front-page evidence of God at work and of their faith affirmed. Thus, most newspapers stressed Father Keating's intervention, publishing all or part of the Associated Press's triptych, which showed him talking to my father, then listening, and finally helping my father to safety.

Then again, the appeal of the story may have suggested a theme even more universal than religion: our need for hope. My father, in the throes of despair, was saved by the most serendipitous of circumstances. Although it's impossible to know whether another individual could've talked my father off the ledge, the man who *was* able to just happened to be walking by at the time and also to be the one chosen, out of a group of three priests, to speak to my father. Perhaps this gives us all reason to hope, even in the bleakest of situations, that a stranger will rescue us as well.

The newspapers editors' choice of photos and captions—"Plunge Thwarted," "Saved—by Words," "Would-Be Suicide"—must have influenced readers' perceptions. Yet, no matter how captioned or cropped, those images remain like their own Rorschach test, of sorts, for each viewer, who can impose their own meaning on them. For the readers in 1957, that significance may have been related to religious or existential themes, or to the political fears and uncertainties of the time, or perhaps even to personal experience. In my case, it had taken more than fifty years to confront what the images meant to me.

EPILOGUE

ON A SATURDAY AFTERNOON THE FOLLOWING SPRING, I drove into town to say goodbye to the owners of the dry cleaners. The business would be under new ownership starting Monday.

On the way, I noticed the two wind turbines that had recently been erected. I'd never seen their blades spinning so rapidly, and I pulled over to see if their whir was as noisy as the neighbors had feared. I turned off the engine and rolled down my window but heard nothing other than the sound of a car passing me from the opposite direction.

As I gazed at the sky, something about its grays reminded me of how it had looked as I drove to the dry cleaners on that Saturday in July, six years earlier. I exhaled. If I'd stopped along the way, the truck would have been long gone by the time I left the dry cleaners, and I would have gotten home safely and gone to that dinner party.

Katie was standing behind the counter when I entered. I looked to my left reflexively. I always liked to check out the selection in her lending library, which usually consisted of ten books or so. I remembered her handing me *The Girl with the Dragon Tattoo* before it had made its big splash. The shelf was now empty.

"I'm so glad I caught you. Is this really your last day?"

"Certainly is. We're heading out of East Hampton on Monday. Sold almost everything and we're heading west in our RV."

"Nice! How long will you be gone?"

"Well, kind of forever, I guess. We've decided to retire and just travel, get jobs as we need them. We might settle somewhere, but only if the place really grabs us."

She looked too young to be retiring; her skin was practically unlined, her forehead uncreased. My jaw might have dropped, because she quickly added, "I'm not as young as you think!"

Apparently not. Maybe her appearance wasn't a reflection of her age, I thought, but of how she'd lived her life—with security, no anxiety. That must be it. But young or not, she was acting on one of my and Ed's fantasies. I couldn't ignore the actual pang of envy I felt in my chest.

"Wow. That's fantastic. Good luck with it all."

"Thanks so much. I think you'll like the new owner. He's a nice guy, likes people."

"Well, I'll have to introduce myself."

Katie smiled. "You won't have to say too much. We've already told him about you."

Katie's husband, George, who had been working by the dryers at the other end of the room, came over to the counter. He, on the other hand, did look old enough to retire, but that might have been the extra weight around his middle.

"Yeah," he said, "he knows all about you."

"Oh God, the squirrel story?"

"Yep," they said in unison.

"And the accident, I guess."

"Of course!" Katie raised her eyebrows and smiled. She looked to her right, through the plate glass window that fronted the street. "I remember that so well. You'd just given us a check, and we'd been laughing about something. Then I walked over to the cash register and heard a thud behind me. I couldn't believe it. I thought you were dead."

"And that's when you ran out, George, right? I remember you."

"Oh, yeah. It was something. You know, the driver, when he got out of the truck, he went and sat on that bench there, the one facing the sidewalk, and just cried . . ."

Perhaps wanting to steer the conversation in a more positive direction, Katie interrupted, "Amy, you were so lucky . . . when I think about what I saw, and then here you are now. It's amazing."

I gave her a hug, but when I noticed the red overspreading George's face, I stuck out my hand and we shook.

I walked down to the curb, and before stepping into the crosswalk, turned and waved. I *had* been lucky. In ways that neither Katie nor anyone else (except for Ed) could ever know.

———

I'd been so careful, I thought, to place myself in stark relief to my father. To do otherwise at the time seemed too dangerous. Any shared ambition or passion could be a carrier gene for mental illness. And so, if my father was too fragile to handle the business world, I would be a lawyer. If my father couldn't support himself, I would be financially independent. If writing caused him persistent blocks, I wouldn't even attempt it. If he struggled with depression, I would force myself to be a pillar of emotional strength. If his vulnerability was splashed across front pages, mine would be buried so deep I could pretend it didn't exist. Those reflexive decisions hadn't created a separate identity, however, but rather a series of stimuli and responses that chained some very deep part of me to him . . . and to my mother.

There had been nothing extraordinary about that dark blue pickup, no special features, nothing to suggest it could uncover a wrinkle in time or my lifelong disguises. Up to that point, I had traveled the territory of my childhood so thoroughly I thought I could find my way through it blindfolded. But after the accident, as if guided at times by the orange of cosmic traffic cones, I found myself taking an unfamiliar detour.

Midway through the crosswalk, I stopped at the sign on the pedestal warning vehicles to stop. I smiled at a man who was walking toward me from the opposite side of the street. He must have wondered why I was standing there. I could see the windshield of an oncoming truck on the empty road. My shoulders dropped. Before the thought could register in my mind, my body remembered the freedom I'd felt as I'd let go of my fear and accepted my vulnerability in the face of that truck.

Since that Saturday, I had regained a sense of freedom (despite my continued resistance) far more profound and lasting than I'd experienced on that crosswalk. I had ended up where it had all begun—on the ledge—and now, for the first time, I really knew myself. It was late in life to start over, but that's where I was . . . where I am. And from here I can see at last the three of us: my father, my mother, and me—our shared vulnerabilities, our distinct selves.

I inhaled. The spring air flowed through me, even into those hiding places where my fear had taken refuge for so long. But I was standing guard no more. And although no longer occupied by fear, those hiding places were still full. Like the air, my compassion filled them effortlessly.

ACKNOWLEDGMENTS

The completion of this book—which started as a thank-you note to a friend—feels like a miracle. Yet this book would have never happened without the enormous amount of support, encouragement, and guidance I received from so many along the way. I'm extremely grateful to:

Patsy (Ribner) Zendel, my eleventh-grade English teacher, for inspiring me to write and for caring so deeply about her students.

Randi Dickson and Joanne Pilgrim, for the early encouragement and guidance that gave me the confidence to continue.

Sarah Saffian, an inspiring author and teacher at the Writing Institute at Sarah Lawrence College, whose early editing and instruction set me on this path.

Cathy Rowe, for her perceptive insights and patient listening as I wrestled with the key question of my book.

Sue Ade, Alan Brody, Sarah Conover, Magda Monteil Davis, Ann Green, Tim Hillegonds, Ann Garretson Marshall, Terry Marshall, Nancy McGlasson, and Dag Scheer, my talented fellow writers at the Iowa Summer Writing Festival in 2015 and the RRWW reunion in 2016, for their patient and thoughtful feedback.

Maryann Calendrille and the members of the Ashawagh Hall Writers' Workshop, for their helpful suggestions on several chapters.

Carol Bandini, Jennifer Cross, Margaret Garsetti, Priscilla Heine, Cristian Majcherski, Nancy Nagle, and Bill Nagle for graciously volunteering to read an early draft and offering their sensitive comments.

Hannah Polauf, for cheerfully coming to my rescue with her technological and design expertise.

The late Nancy Nagle Kelley, who, despite the formidable challenges she faced, generously found the strength to read my manuscript and offer encouragement.

Jacquelyn Gavron, for her astute comments, sharp editing, and patient good humor as I struggled through multiple drafts.

Nancy McGlasson (again), an "adopted" cousin, for commenting on a chunk of my manuscript when she could have spent that time on her own wonderful writing.

Adam Osterweil, for the laser focus (tinged with humor) he so generously trained on my final drafts.

Hope Edelman, an exceptional author, teacher, and coach, for her keen observations, creative instruction, brilliant suggestions, and patient insistence to, as my father always counseled, go deeper.

Brooke Warner, Shannon Green, Krissa Lagos, and the entire team at She Writes Press, for taking on this first-time author.

Publicist Caitlin Hamilton Summie and her team for getting my memoir out to readers.

My acupuncturist, whose gentle methods of healing and trauma resolution created the conditions that allowed my story to emerge.

My brother Jim Turner, for his profound understanding and wisdom.

My sister, Louise Stinespring, for her unparalleled support

and encouragement, even as she faced her own challenges. I so wish she had lived to see this book's publication.

My parents, Harold M. Turner Jr. and Virginia B. Turner, and my brother Harold Turner. I hope they know this book was written out of love for them.

My sons, Matthew and Peter, for, each in their own way, wholeheartedly supporting my writing—which, as I know from personal experience, can be complicated for a child to do.

My husband, Ed, for whom—even after all I've learned about writing—I am still at a loss when it comes to expressing the depth of my gratitude. Simply put, without his encouragement, patience, understanding, and love, there would be no book.

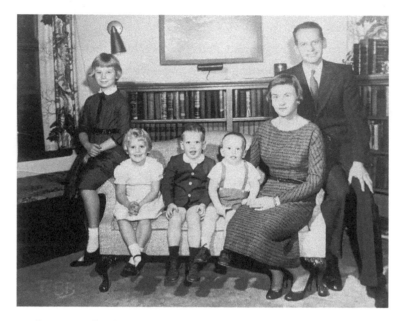

The Turner family in November 1957, sometime within the two weeks
before my father climbed onto the ledge

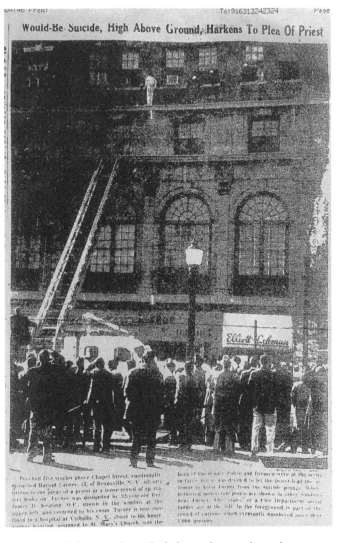

Would-Be Suicide, High Above Ground, Harkens To Plea Of Priest

Perched five stories above Chapel Street, emotionally disturbed Harold Turner, 43, of Bronxville, N. Y. silently listens to the pleas of a priest as a tense crowd of spectators looks on. Turner was dissuaded by 32-year-old Rev. James D. Keating, O.P., shown in the window at the upper left, and returned to his room. Turner is now confined to a hospital at Valhalla, N. Y., closer to his home. Father Keating, assigned to St. Mary's Church, was the hero of the drama. Police and firemen were at the scene in force. Later it was decided to let the priest lead the attempt to keep Turner from the suicide plunge. White-helmeted motorcycle police are shown in other windows near Turner. The "stairs" of a Fire Department aerial ladder are at the left. In the foreground is part of the crowd of curious which eventually numbered more than 1,000 persons.

My father stands on the ledge as the crowd watches

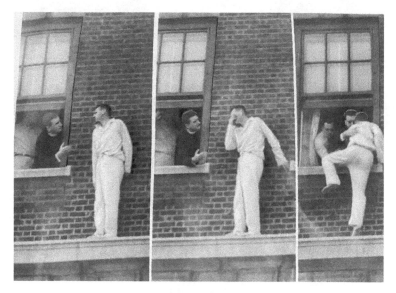

Father Keating and my father

ABOUT THE AUTHOR

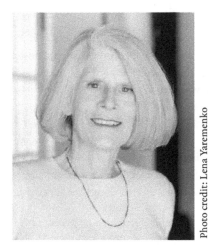

Photo credit: Lena Yaremenko

AMY TURNER was born in Bronxville, New York. She holds a degree in political science from Boston University and a Juris Doctor from New York Law School. After practicing law (rather unhappily) for twenty-two years, she finally found the courage to change careers at forty-eight and become a (very happy) seventh-grade social studies teacher. A long-time meditator and avid reader who loves to swim and bike, Amy lives in East Hampton, New York, with her husband, Ed, to whom she's been married for forty years, and their dog, Fred. Amy and Ed have two sons. *On the Ledge* is Amy's first book.

SELECTED TITLES FROM SHE WRITES PRESS

She Writes Press is an independent publishing company founded to serve women writers everywhere. Visit us at www.shewritespress.com.

A Different Kind of Same: A Memoir by Kelley Clink. $16.95, 978-1-63152-999-3. Several years before Kelley Clink's brother hanged himself, she attempted suicide by overdose. In the aftermath of his death, she traces the evolution of both their illnesses, and wonders: If he couldn't make it, what hope is there for her?

Patchwork: A Memoir of Love and Loss by Mary Jo Doig. $16.95, 978-1-63152-449-3. Part mystery and part inspirational memoir, *Patchwork* chronicles the riveting healing journey of one woman who, following the death of a relative, has a flashback that opens a dark passageway back to her childhood and the horrific secrets that have long been buried deep inside her psyche.

Rethinking Possible: A Memoir of Resilience by Rebecca Faye Smith Galli. $16.95, 978-1-63152-220-8. After her brother's devastatingly young death tears her world apart, Becky Galli embarks upon a quest to recreate the sense of family she's lost—and learns about healing and the transformational power of love over loss along the way.

The Tell: A Memoir by Linda I. Meyers. $16.95, 978-1-63152-355-7. Meyers's account of losing her mother to suicide when she was twenty-eight—and of how, determined to give the death meaning, she changed her own life for the better.

The Strongbox: Searching for My Absent Father by Terry Sue Harms. $16.95, 978-1-63152-775-3. Following the unexpected death of her alcoholic mother, sixteen-year-old Terry Sue decides her biological father, whom she doesn't know, could change her life for the better. By the time she finally finds him, however—after decades of searching—she understands that she has cultivated the nurturing she craved from him for herself.

Where Have I Been All My Life? A Journey Toward Love and Wholeness by Cheryl Rice. $16.95, 978-1-63152-917-7. Rice's universally relatable story of how her mother's sudden death launched her on a journey into the deepest parts of grief—and, ultimately, toward love and wholeness.